THE ULTRA MARATHON BIBLE

YOUR #1 BEGINNER'S TRAINING GUIDE TO PREPARE,
RUN, AND SURVIVE YOUR FIRST 50K TO 100
MILE RACE

SAMUEL NASH

CONTENTS

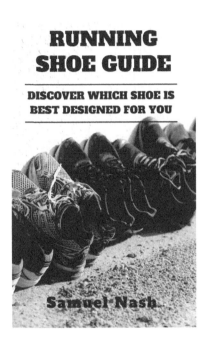

This running shoe guide goes into detail about the many different types of running shoes, and which one is the best fit for you.

INTRODUCTION

I fell in love with running when I was in high school. I was overweight, and my family told me what I already knew. I needed to make a change in my life, so I began with the basics. I ate healthier, exercised, and watched my weight. But it wasn't until I signed up for my high school track and field team that I really felt my life change.

Over the next decade, I ran more and more. I started with a few miles, then several 5ks, and then moved up to 10ks. After that, I ran half marathons and eventually moved up to marathons. I was hooked. I've remained so ever since. When I found out about Ultra Marathons–races longer than traditional marathons–I knew I had to try them.

I didn't think it was possible, but Ultra Marathons made me fall in love with running all over again. Over the past few years, I've run several Ultra Marathons and have enjoyed (almost) every minute of it. The training, the race, and most of all, the high you get from challenging yourself and achieving your goals are all beautiful parts of this experience.

I know what it's like to think you'd never be able to complete even one mile. It's hard, and the idea of an Ultra Marathon seems impossible. But completing the race is possible. It's possible for anyone to do, as long as you are willing to put in the time and be patient with yourself. Anyone can go from not being able to run even one mile to running one hundred miles.

EVERY PERSON RUNS MARATHONS

It may seem impossible right now, but the truth is that everyone runs marathons. For some of us, these marathons manifest in the form of long hours in the office with the goal of bringing home enough money for our families. For others, a marathon means going from work to home, to soccer practice, to music practice, to the grocery store, and back home. Still, others stay up late for hours upon hours on end, studying hard for an exam that will take place the next day. Do you see? You already have the mindset of a marathon runner.

The only difference with a running marathon is that the race takes place in a physical and mental arena. Ultra Marathons require you to push yourself beyond what you thought you were capable of accomplishing. They require preparation, practice, and resilience. But isn't that life?

The feelings we have about new challenges are the same no matter what arena they're in. Anytime we begin a new journey into a place that we've never been before, we feel the same apprehension. After all, life is full of unexpected things, and no matter how much we prepare or think we're ready, there always seems to be a new surprise. Yet, we learn to grow and adapt. After we see that we are able to handle this thing, we may even start to feel confident.

Think about the first time you went to a new school. Maybe your experience was positive or not so much. Whatever the result, if you're reading this book, you got through it, and you survived. Despite the apprehension, the challenges, and the difficulty of learning a new social and educational world, you got through it. You reaped the benefits of your experience, endured the hard things, and pushed forward.

What I really want you to understand is that when you are training for an Ultra Marathon, you aren't doing anything that you have not already done. You know what it feels like to be out of breath. You know what it feels like to train and prepare in order to reach a goal. You know what it feels like to mentally steel yourself for something challenging. This isn't scary. You've done this before.

The goal of this Ultra Marathon Bible is to take all of those previous experiences and use them to help you accomplish your next big goal, running and finishing an Ultra Marathon. Following these instructions will help you design the best path forward. We'll be starting from the very beginning and running through all the way to the end. From the moment you decide that you want to run an Ultra Marathon, all the way to the moment where you cross the finish line and raise your arms in victory.

We will explore all the highs and exciting things to look forward to during training and on race day. We will also take time to discuss the difficulties and realities involved in taking on the Ultra Marathon challenge. Hang in there and believe in yourself. Don't worry; we'll do this together.

TO THE RUNNER

If you're someone like me and you've already found your love for running, then maybe this is the next big step for you. If you have run 5ks and 10ks already and you want to challenge yourself, then look no further. If this is not your first rodeo and you've run long races before, welcome to the world of Ultra Marathons, the next step in your running evolution.

An Ultra Marathon is going to be very different from the races you've had up to this point. This race will challenge you in ways you may not have considered before. But if you're here, it's because you love running. That love will empower you to overcome obstacles and push past boundaries. A runner must do what they were made to do. They must move quickly past brush and bramble over asphalt and concrete.

When asked why she was running, Annie, from the 2014 movie of the same name, said it best. "It gets me to places quicker."

We love the feeling of getting to places 'quicker' and the experience of the journey between point A and point B. The feeling of our feet hitting the pavement in that steady cadence. Running makes us come alive. Races are just a different way to experience that life. Ultra Marathons are just a different way to experience races.

Whatever the reason you've decided to pick up this book, know that you're not just holding a set of instructions. You are holding a kindred spirit. This book contains the heart of a runner and the passion that comes with it. As we journey through the process of considering, preparing, training, and participating in an Ultra Marathon, take time to enjoy the process. Don't just read the instructions and do what I say (although that's an excellent way to make progress). Feel what each of these sections means to you and for you. Think about the time, investments, effort, and care you are putting into this experience.

Now, go do it.

1

WHERE TO BEGIN?

If you don't think you were born to run, you're not only denying history. You're denying who you are.

— CHRISTOPHER MCDOUGALL

Running has been around just as long as man has. Over the course of our history, we were expert runners, lost that knowledge, gained it again, and now we're perfecting the art. The more we learn about our bodies and the science behind their physiology, the better we become at mastering athletics and sports. Even if you don't fully believe, trust me —we were designed to run.

WE WERE DESIGNED TO RUN

It seems like, from the beginning of time, we were designed to be able to run. From the structure of our bones to the ability our body has to adapt quickly, we are inexplicably shaped in a way that optimizes running. In fact, we are one of the few animals that can run at a steady pace for several miles and consciously train ourselves to do so.

When you look at the body and how it's constructed, one of the first things that stands out as different from other animals is the way that we consume oxygen. While we share a similar lung structure with other mammalian creatures on this planet, no other creature consumes oxygen the way humans do. The structure of our bodies, the location of our lungs, the placement of our nose and mouth, and the use of both our breathing and sweat glands to help control body temperature are all part of a system designed to optimize the use of oxygen. Not only do we use oxygen to live, but also to break down glucose and provide energy for our bodies. What an efficient process!

However, our design for running doesn't end there. We have also developed physically to maximize our capacity for running. Several studies by professionals have noted that our muscles and bones seem to be arranged in such a way that they are perfect for long-distance running. Not only are our legs the strongest parts of our bodies, but they also have several muscles that play a role in stabilizing the rest of the body during extended use.

For example, take a look at the **gluteus maximus**—your butt. This muscle is one of the largest and most powerful muscles that we have in our body. Not only does it provide additional force when it comes to walking, but the muscle also stabilizes our torso and upper body as we trot along. Sure, we don't actually use this muscle as much when we are just walking, but the gluteus maximus really kicks in and becomes fully engaged when we are running.

We also sweat much differently than other animals on the planet. Although many different animals sweat through their skin (monkeys, horses, etc.), we are one of the few creatures on this earth with over **2 million sweat glands** and the ability to release moisture in such significant amounts to cool off. If you think about a large machine constructed to work on intense or heavy project, there has to be a way to vent built-up energy in the form of heat or steam.

You can compare the human body to a steam engine that regularly exhausts smoke and moisture as it chugs along down the railway. In a lot of ways, our bodies are exactly like that. As we work, we heat up, and we expel that heat with moisture and sweat to cool us down and keep us running efficiently and from getting overheated. A steam engine was designed to keep moving forward along the rails. We were designed to run.

There are two main phases to typical human running. The first phase is called **stance,** and the second phase is called **swing.** During stance, your heel hits the ground, and you move forward until your toe pushes off of the ground and propels you straight ahead. That is the end of the stance portion of the cycle.

The second part of the cycle is the swing. This part of the cycle involves your foot going aerial and swinging forward. The cycle is complete once your foot hits the ground again, beginning the next stance cycle. The running cycle consists of alternating swing and stance over and over. Like the rest of our body, our feet have also adapted to optimize this process.

Not only do we have a sturdy **calcaneus** bone in our heel, but we also have very springy tendons and ligaments that help to absorb the force of our foot connecting with the ground and generating more energy to move forward. Notice how your big toe is the straightest and most prominent digit on your foot.

Your big toe plays a prominent role in helping you maintain your balance and optimize the end of the stance cycle. Your big toe is often the last part of your foot to leave the ground during running.

Still not convinced? Why don't you compare us to other animals on the face of this earth? There are dozens, if not hundreds, of animals that are much faster when it comes to running. Many of these animals have optimized ligaments, muscles, and fast-twitch fibers that allow them to cover the distance in a very short amount of time. But very few animals have muscles that allow them to run an endurance race. Most animals will clearly outrun us in short distances. But humans have been using their endurance-built strength for thousands of years.

One of the earliest and most notable uses for our endurance build was basic hunting. Although humans are not the fastest nor the strongest of all the creatures on this earth, we have used our intelligence and our ability to endure and persist to our advantage. In fact, unlike cheetahs which will go after a large herd of animals and run them down quickly, humans will track animals, tiring them out until the animal is so fatigued that it can no longer run and escape. The human can then claim their prize. We see this even now. Well, before we learned how to cultivate, farm, and raise animals as livestock, we were hunting and tracking creatures. Studies of bushmen and native Indians have revealed a lot about the way we used to stalk prey for one to two days in order to tire and capture them.

UNDERSTANDING THE ULTRA MARATHON

So what does all this have to do with the Ultra Marathon? Well, in order to fathom the incredible physical trial that is the Ultra Marathon, you need to understand first that it is entirely possible for you to run an Ultra Marathon. You were designed to run. The Ultra Marathon can often be intimidating if you've never run long races before. Chances are, if you are reading this book, you're interested in either setting a very far-off goal for running, or you've been running for a while and are trying to learn how to reach the next level. In order to do this, we need to first under-stand what the Ultra Marathon is.

The Ultra Marathon, simply put, is any race longer than a marathon (26.2 miles) (42.2 km). Commonly, these races start at 50k (31.1 miles) (50 km) and can go well beyond 100 miles (161 km). But that is by no means the cap. In fact, the longest Ultra Marathon is the **Sri Chinmoy Self Transcendence** 3100 mile (4989 km) race. This race takes around 52 days to complete, and people often run from 6 AM to midnight.

Ultra Marathons are the ultimate test of running endurance and require a lot of training in order to meet the challenges. The first Ultra Marathon challenges were actually walking challenges. Men would see how far they could walk in a day and would often make bets on the amount of distance. Over time, this evolved into running, and now we have people who may run for multiple days at a time, stopping only to sleep and eat.

These multiple-day challenges are called stage races. Usually, they are the races that go for 100 miles or more. The idea is that the runner will complete a certain amount of distance for each stage. And at the end of the stage, they will then have the opportunity to rest and recuperate. For some Ultra Marathons, this means that the person at the end of the day makes camp. For others, this means that the person will be able to stay in a luxury hotel where they can rest and put their feet up.

There are also 'time' Ultra Marathons. And these usually range from anywhere between 6 to 12 hours of running. Typically these are different from stage marathons in that they involve the person running a shorter loop and logging the time and distance that they complete the loop in the required time. The 3100 mile (4989 km) race that I mentioned before is an example of a time-based Ultra Marathon. Marathons like this allow people to stop and rest as needed and get whatever nutrients or hydration their body requires to keep going. The loops are generally shorter, and the focus is on completing the distance in the time required more so than advancing through the different stages of the race.

Sounds pretty cool, right? You may, at this point, be feeling pretty pumped up and excited to experience such a challenge. The idea of seeing various locales and advancing through stages to set up camp or experience a luxurious hotel at the end of each day can be a very seductive vision. Or maybe your blood starts pumping by just being able to do what you love - run and achieve your goal in the shortest amount of time you can. And that's good.

However, one of the things that you need to remember is that you cannot immediately go from a marathon to an Ultra. Even if you are an experienced runner, it takes time, training, and preparation to run an Ultra Marathon. New runners especially need to ease into long-distance races. Although your body is *designed* for long-distance running, it may not be *conditioned* for it yet.

That is where training and preparation come in. But first, you'll need to determine what your goal is and which race is best for you.

PICKING YOUR RACE

Making decisions is hard. Whether you are trying to decide between apples and oranges, between two fast-food restaurants, clothing brands, or whether you should train or not, making a decision means that you are risking making the wrong one. We, as humans, always seem to want to make the right decision. But, we struggle. Sometimes we let our emotions get ahead of us, and sometimes we try to do the 'logical' thing and end up hurting ourselves in the process.

Indecision is usually the result of fear and a lack of knowledge. Coincidentally, the more you know, the more confident you can make a decision. Right now, you may be looking at the Ultra Marathon world and feeling somewhat lost. That's okay, that's normal. The best way to combat this feeling is to learn more about the different options you have and how to determine what will work best for you. In this next section, we will explore all the different elements you need to consider when choosing your next race.

Canadian educator Laurence J. Peter said, "If you don't know where you are going, you will probably end up somewhere else."

This is especially true for runners, both physically and figuratively. As you get ready to train and learn more about the kind of race that you want to run, you need to first identify what your goal is. The race you want to run depends on the distance you're willing to go as well as the time and intensity of the race that you are pursuing.

Once you've identified the kind of race, you need to get to know the race. This means understanding the qualifications, the characteristics, and many other factors. Identifying and understanding the race gives you the tools and understanding to pick your ideal race and make a potentially overwhelming and discouraging experience into a positive one that you will never forget.

Which Race is Best For You?

Determining which race is best for you starts with figuring out the distance that you want to run. As mentioned earlier, new runners should start off with shorter distances and slowly increase them. However, that might also be the case for seasoned runners who are not used to the long and vigorous challenges of running a multiple-day race. In either case, runners need to be patient with themselves as they get acclimated to a new type of running.

Most runners will be best served if they begin with a standard 50k. This is an excellent introduction to long-distance running because it's a closer race to a standard marathon. In fact, it's only adding on 4.8 miles (7.7 km). This seems a lot more achievable than a 62.1 mile (100km). It also means that if you've already run a marathon, you'll only need to do a little more preparation to get to the 50k mark.

On average, every time you increase your racing distance, you should add on an estimated **six months** of preparation to get race-ready. Depending on how many extra miles you are adding to your previous race, you may even need to add on more. Jumping from a standard 26.2 mile (42.2 km) marathon to a 62 mile (100k) marathon is a pretty big leap. You are adding over 35 miles to your race. Depending on your training schedule, an extra six months might not be enough. There's nothing wrong with taking your time. In fact, it's encouraged. Jumping into a race that you have not given adequate time in training for is dangerous and can be very demotivating.

Most Ultras are broken down into distances of 50k, 100k, 50 miles, and 100 miles. Anything beyond this is more of a custom challenge. For a 50k, you'll need to have about six months of preparation. The same goes for a 100k; however, the preparation and training will be more intense if you have not run a 50k before the 100k. For a 50 mile run, you should choose a race that is six months out if you have running experience, but you'll need more than just six months if you don't have any running experience. In fact, you should shoot for something under 50 miles if you don't have experience running long distances at all. 100 mile races are no joke, and you'll need time to prepare unless you are already an elite Ultra runner. For a 100 mile race, you should choose a race that is at least six months out, if not more, to be ready.

Picking the right race for you also means understanding yourself. What is your purpose for running this race? Are you looking for a race that allows you to get a little exercise? Are you looking for a race that will create opportunities for you to make friends and develop your social circle? What about a race that helps you strengthen the bonds of friendship you already have? Are you hoping to find something that will test your limits? Or are you just trying something new? Answering these questions can help you determine which race you need to run. Also, knowing how much preparation, time, and money you can afford to spend on this race will give you a better idea of which race is ideal.

Before you even step foot on the course, you should be evaluating your own motives. Why do you want to run an Ultra Marathon? If you are not fully committed to this race or only have a passing interest in it, you'll probably not be able to finish. Races require commitment and lots of effort. Runners train for months—in some cases, years. Out of respect for the sport and the other participants—most of all yourself—make sure you are entering your race with the proper expectations and motivations.

You should also take some time to know your body. Although we were all created to run, some seem to have an easier time than others. Even though we were all designed to speak, some people speak easier and more clearly than others. The same is true with running. If you know that you have always struggled with running, you can improve with training and practice. But it may take more time, and you may need to start with a race that is simpler. There is nothing wrong with that. You will eventually get to the point where you can run any race you'd like. But knowing your body and your history can help you to pick the correct race up front and avoid disappointment and embarrassment. This simple reflection can be the difference between a runner finishing a race and tapping out within the first mile.

Don't forget about the external factors of the race that drew you to the idea in the first place. Every race seems to carry its own personality. Think about what your goals and objectives are for your race and find a race that matches those. For example, are you a hard-core runner and looking to get the best time possible? Or are you just looking to finish the race but have an opportunity to see some beautiful scenic views along the way? Do you want to race with hundreds of spectators and crowds cheering? Or do you prefer something quieter where you can get lost in your thoughts and just enjoy the solitude of nature? Not only will your answers to some of these questions tell you more about yourself, but they can also reveal the best race for you at this point in time. When picking a race, don't neglect your own goals and objectives.

Getting to Know Your Race

Understanding the race you'll be running is a lot like learning to understand another person. You build a relationship by asking questions and expressing interest in that person. Throughout the course of getting to know someone, you are constantly comparing their perspective to yours. This allows you to find places where you have things in common and where you differ.

In many relationships, we decide whether the relationship will progress forward by whether or not we have things in common and how bothered we are by the things we don't have in common. In many ways, the same is true for getting to know and selecting your race. You'll need to ask questions to get more information about what the race entails. You'll need to compare what's important to you to what the race offers. Then you'll need to evaluate if this race has enough of the things that you want in order to be worth your time and effort. If there are too many red flags—things that bother you about the race—it's probably not the right one for you. Let the race go; there will be others.

Getting to know your race is also one of the most critical parts of the training process. You'll need to know everything from the altitude you'll be running to how much the race costs. Ultra Marathons require a lot of preparation, not just in the physical training but also in the planning. Let's go through a few factors that you want to consider as you seek to understand your race.

Altitude and elevation play a vital role in how you train to prepare for a race. Higher elevation and altitude mean that not only is the air colder, but it also contains fewer oxygen molecules. In addition, the pressure outside of your body is lower than inside your body, so it's difficult to draw in the air that you need, and the air that you do draw in is less dense with oxygen. This means your body has to be even more efficient with how it pumps blood and the oxygen in the blood throughout your system. Yes, it's just as complex as it sounds. Your body is a machine, and you need to make sure that your machine is optimized for the task it's been given. Knowing your altitude and elevation beforehand can tell you whether or not a race is for you as well as whether or not you should train at higher elevations in order to be ready for the race.

Another environmental challenge to keep an eye on is the **terrain** that you'll be running on. What kind of ground does the race path cover? Is it gravel? Concrete? Dirt? What percentage of the trail is made up of these different kinds of terrain? Will you be expected to cross rivers or other bodies of water? Will you be in a location with lots of shade or a location where you can be exposed to high sun rays? All of these little factors can play a role in how well you perform. If you train in a shady environment for six months just to find out that you're running along the highway where there are no trees or shade, you may have all of the conditioning you need, but the heat will sap your strength. In addition to this, the light intensity may mess with your mind to the point where you don't even want to complete the race anymore. Therefore, it's good practice to run races only in terrain that you have accessible to you. If you're used to running on grass and flat surfaces, then jagged ground and loose gravel may be challenging.

Along those lines, the **environment and climate** play a large role in how you run. As mentioned before, if you're in locations that have a lot of sun or locations where there's a high likelihood of rain, knowing your environment can help you plan ahead. Sometimes something as simple as climate or the weather can make or break an Ultra runner. By monitoring the climate and the weather, you can help to stay on top of what the worst-case scenario may be and prepare accordingly. Knowing that your race takes place in the rainy season of the location you plan to run means that not only do you need to bring the proper rain gear, but you need to practice running in wet and slippery environments.

Make an effort to know what your **start time** is and the **time of day** that you'll be running. Not only is planning ahead important in order to avoid events like anniversaries and other festivities, but you also need to know so that you allow for adequate time to prepare. Not to mention the time of day you begin can drastically impact your race's success. Knowing that you'll be running at night means that you need reflective and illumination gear. This also means that you need to understand and experience what it's like running in the dark.

Keep in mind that Ultra Marathons vary in **attendance and popularity**. Knowing the race that you are planning to attend means knowing how many people are also registering. Some races are booked out many months before the actual race. Other races don't really have a cap and tend to be more of a cattle-style lurch down the path. Then other races have meager attendance and sometimes can be lonely to run. Whatever you're looking for, take some time to read and do your due diligence so that you know how many people you can estimate will be in attendance and how far in advance you'll be able to register to get a spot. The cost of an event also might increase or decrease depending on its popularity. Make sure that you're keeping track of the cost and any early bird or late penalties for last-minute cancellations.

While you're planning on registering, this is also an excellent time to get an idea of the **rules** and to see if pacers and/or a crew team are allowed. Some races allow you to bring people along to help you keep your pace or get through really tough moments, while other races insist that you run solo and don't allow extra people on the trail with you. This is something that you'll need to determine beforehand so that you can plan accordingly or, if you absolutely need someone, skip the race altogether. Make sure that whatever race you are committing to, you are comfortable with. Read the rules, ask questions, and plan accordingly.

2

FOUR KEY ELEMENTS IN ANY ULTRA PROGRAM

Training and preparation are essential to success in any running program, but especially when trying to compete in an Ultra. These races tend to be so intense that a lack of preparation is enough to sideline you completely. While there are a great number of things you should consider when planning and training for an Ultra, there are four main elements that will drastically impact your success. Your **training, nutrition, hydration, and recovery** are vital components of how you run an Ultra.

There are many things you have to do to prepare for an Ultra that will make your life much easier. However, many of those things can be compromised without completely taking you out of the race. These four elements must be practiced in order for you to continue to participate in Ultra Marathon races. Without them, your body will fail, and your dreams and ambitions to run a good race will not come to fruition.

TRAINING

This may seem obvious, but you cannot complete a race you have not trained for. Your body is just not in the suitable condition to handle the stress of the intense activity you put your body through. Not only do you risk injury without proper training, but you risk wasting money, time, and opportunity. So many people have given up on the joys of running because they did not prepare adequately. Instead of finding someone who could coach them or following a training plan, they ran a few miles a couple of times a week and expected to be able to manage over 30 miles.

You have to train if you want to be successful. If you're not willing to put in the time and work to make your body ready, then you might want to find a different activity to pursue. Ultra marathons are for those who want to improve. There's no better way to improve than to practice and hone your body to peak condition in order to handle the rigors of the trail ahead.

Training not only prepares your body for the race but also boosts your confidence in your abilities. As you train, you'll see your improvement and realize that you are capable of doing more today than you were last week. This confidence is important, and we will talk more about mindset later in this book. But for now, it's important to note that confidence helps you stay motivated and encourages you to pursue your goal, no matter the trials.

In order to train successfully, you need a solid training plan. This training plan can differ from person to person, but there are some basic concepts you should always hold onto. Understanding *how* to plan, the 80/20 rule, and how different runs are structured can help you feel more confident in your running and prepare you for the challenge ahead.

Planning for Success

Planning is essential for any level of success. The key to a successful race is a solid training plan. A training plan gives you the guidance that you need in order to be successful in your marathon goal. A good training plan will build you up gradually, allowing your body opportunities to rest and recuperate while also pushing it past its current limits. Your plan should be well calculated, thought out, and built towards the goal that you wish to accomplish.

In this book, I have included training plans for 50k, 50mi, 100k, and 100mi races. These training programs are just guidelines to follow. You can use them or find another reliable program online in order to take your first steps towards Ultra Marathon training. Make sure that the plan that you select is based on your current ability and meets the time frame that you wish to be ready for your race. Also, make sure the plan is based on the 10% rule.

The 10% rule is a guide that most professional and elite runners follow to safely maintain steady progress. The 10% rule states that you should only increase your training by 10% at most each week. This will help prevent injury and allow you to set realistic goals. Your body does best with a slow and steady increase in activity so that it can adapt to the stress of the new performance. Since you may not have done this before, you'll have to be gentle and patient as your system acclimates. Don't rush; that will only lead to injury and setbacks.

As a general milestone, you should be running around 20-30 miles a week for a 50K race, 35-40 miles a week for a 50 mi race, 40-45 miles for a 100K, and 50 miles a week for a 100 mile race. While these numbers can be tweaked and adjusted to meet your needs, they present an outline of what it takes in order to complete each of these races.

While these provide a very good outline for various marathon races, it's important to note that Ultra training plans may differ a bit from normal marathon plans. One of the most significant differences will be that speed is not as important in Ultra Marathons because of the longer distances. You end up training for fatigue and endurance more than trying to maximize your speed at various points during the race. Ultra Marathons also require you to train your mind to endure the extended strain on your body.

The 80/20 Rule

The **80/20** rule is a fundamental rule to be aware of and follow. Basically, you need to make sure that your easy training days stay easy so that you can work harder on the hard days. The 80/20 rule states that runners should focus on spending 80% of their weekly training at a low to moderate intensity and 20% at a moderate to high intensity. This is a structure that's followed by many top-level endurance athletes, including cyclists, swimmers, and triathletes.

Of course, this makes the 80/20 rule a particularly good rule for runners who are trying to train for an Ultra Marathon. Not only that, but the 80/20 rule can be used for any level of race, even if you are just trying to run a 5k. This structure helps prevent you from over-training while still adequately preparing your body for the performance stress ahead.

The challenge of this rule is that you have to pay very close attention to how you run. You will need to know what an easy or moderate pace is for you, how much you're running in a week, and the distance you can run in a set amount of time. The truth is that high-intensity training will not give you the endurance you need to complete longer races like marathons. That means you need to intersperse that training with low-intensity training that focuses on extending the amount of time you're able to maintain a slower pace.

Of course, to do this means that you need to be able to figure out what your intensity level is. Many specialists break intensity down into **zones**. Often, zone one will be equivalent to a warm-up or cool-down jog, and zone five will be an intense uphill run. In between are zones two through four, which mark gradual increases in intensity.

Your intensity can be determined by both your pace as well as your heart rate. As in many gyms, when you can determine your active heart rate, the amount of calories you're burning, or the increased work your lungs are putting in, you can get an idea of the current intensity of your workout. You can also determine intensity by finding your baseline pace. This means running at what feels natural for a determined amount of time or distance. Then, aim to beat that time or cover that distance in less time to increase intensity.

How you split up the 80/20 is entirely up to you and, if you have one, your coach. Most of the time, people will just break up their weekly run. For example, if you usually run 50 miles a week, then you will run 40 miles at low to moderate intensity and 10 miles at moderate to high intensity. That means you may run 2 miles for five days that are at a higher intensity than all the other mileage you're putting in.

Now, it will probably be very difficult to run two miles straight at high intensity, especially if you are just beginning your training. Breaking it down into a warm-up, a workout, and a cool-down helps you organize your run in a way that makes sense and is attainable. There is nothing helpful about setting unreasonable expectations.

Running Structure

Running structure is essential to your training plan because it tells you how you will be training and helps runners to better understand various training designs. All training plans will be structured with these types of training exercises, so they need to be understood clearly.

Easy runs are the most common. In fact, the majority of runs that you make will be considered easy. Remember, the easy runs are what will build up your aerobic training, which in turn will allow you to run faster and longer. Even though they may not feel as intense, they are an essential part of the hard work you'll be doing.

Long runs are important, but only so much as they begin to show how far you are from your goal. Once a week, long runs allow you to prepare for race day. Learning to spend time on your feet is crucial, so your body gets used to that sensation.

Tempo runs need to be implemented once a week to help train your body to keep a race pace. While you may not always do this as a beginner Ultra runner, it's meant to help your body get used to maintaining a desired pace for each mile of the race. For Ultra Marathons, it can be very difficult to keep a solid pace per mile. But if this is not your first race or you are planning on competing or beating a previous time, then tempo runs are a very helpful practice. For your first Ultra run, focus on getting the mileage, not so much the pace.

Trail runs are only essential if you know your race will be done mainly on a trail. This is an integral part of that research phase mentioned in Chapter 1, where you'll be looking into and getting to know your race. If you are on a trail for most of your race, you need to make sure you are getting time spent running on trails. It's a very different experience than running on a solid road. You'll have to consistently look at the trail to make sure you are not tripping on roots, rocks, branches, mud, or any other obstruction. This takes practice and experience. In addition, your pace will be slower on a trail due to the different terrain. The more you run different kinds of trails, the better prepared you will be for race day.

Night runs are another type of run that is very different from what you may be used to. Although the track may be the same, there is an art to running at night. Many races don't take place during the night, but if yours does, make sure to practice running without much light.

The **rate of perceived effort (RPE)** is a scale used to identify the intensity of your exercise based on how hard you feel (perceive) your effort to be. This scale can be used for each one of your runs. Your easy runs will be measured based on your RPE as well as your long runs. Your RPE is much more important than maintaining a certain pace per mile. In fact, your RPE can often dictate your pace per mile.

For an easy run (class 1-3), you can still carry on a conversation comfortably, and your breathing is controlled. At a moderate run (class 4-6), you are still somewhat comfortable and can talk, but you're working harder. At a hard run (class 7-9), talking is difficult. You are outside your comfort zone, and breathing is hard. Finally, at max effort (class 10), you are giving it your all. Talking is impossible, and you are struggling to breathe.

Understanding these running structures and determining your RPE sets the foundation for your training plan. Use these techniques to diversify your training and maximize its effectiveness.

NUTRITION

What you put in your body is as equally important, if not more important, than how you train your body. The quality of the fuel you put into a machine directly impacts how well it runs. Your body is no different. Spend time researching different recipes and types of food you can eat. Use this opportunity to learn some new dishes—or how to cook, period. This is training, after all. Training is all about growth and learning.

What better way to supplement your physical training than to grow your culinary ability as well?

Runners are often tempted to neglect nutrition because of the amount they're exercising and the number of calories being burned. The idea that you can eat whatever you want without consequence because your metabolism is high is faulty. Your body will certainly require more calories than usual during training. Paying attention to what goes into your body is even more critical during this period than ever.

Eating to Train

During your training, you'll need to eat a balanced meal of proteins, fats, and carbohydrates. New runners often like to eat like bodybuilders with high protein and low sugars and fats because it seems healthier. But this can be detrimental to your performance. Eating a low-carb diet and running 30, 40, or 50 miles a week is not safe, and eventually, you'll feel it. I know this first hand because I tried that method as well. I ended up burning way more each day than I was eating. It made me feel lightheaded, and my body did not recover from training as fast. It also affected my mood, which didn't help my mental state when training and preparing for race day.

Not only do you need to develop a training plan for eating a balanced diet, but you'll also need to learn to eat and run on your long runs. During your Ultra, you will be running for hours. There will be moments when you can stop and eat a quick and simple meal. But if you want to keep your momentum and maintain a decent pace, you'll be expected to get comfortable with snacking while running.

I also recommend testing your foods and gels before race day so that you won't get sick on your run from a surprise reaction to a new food you just tried. Test how your body responds to sweet, savory, and salty foods. Do the same for all of your drink options as well. Make a short list of foods you like so that you know if you see it at the race, it will work for you.

Again, think of your body as a machine. If you put bad fuel into your machine, it may run, but it's going to die faster and possibly not start again. The same is with your nutrition. Learn how to eat the proper fuel and determine what you need before the run so that during the run, you are operating at maximum output and don't have to worry about finding something that works for you.

The Art of Carb Loading

Carb loading is an art. This practice can help decrease fatigue and increase performance during your race. You're going to want to eat more carbs in the days leading up to your race. This will help your body store more fuel for race day. I know this seems counterintuitive. You'd think that you might want to be lighter or eat less in order to feel better while running. But you absolutely need that energy in order to make it through the race.

A good practice is to cut back on foods that are rich in fats so that you can focus on bringing in more carbs. Whole grains are often recommended when carb loading. These include quinoa and even steel-cut oats. For quality carb-loading, you may end up eating 2.3 to 5.5 grams of carbs per pound every day.

The purpose of carb-loading is to increase the amount of glycogen you hold in order to store up energy. You can't do this by eating a giant dinner the night before the marathon. You have to build up to this, slowly increasing the number of carbs that you are ingesting until you get to around 70% of your caloric intake as being just carbs. This usually takes place around one to three days before the race. However, that increase should also be taking place over time in the week leading up to your race. You don't need to overeat because most training plans have you decreasing the amount of training that you'll be doing as you approach race day anyways.

Take time to learn how to carb load correctly. So many runners make critical mistakes when they try to carb load. Many wait until the night before to load their plate up with a whole bunch of carbs hoping that the food will carry over into the next day and give them the energy they need to get through the race. But all that does is make you feel sluggish and tired in the morning.

As mentioned before, many people have the idea that carb loading is the same thing as what bodybuilders call dirty bulking. This typically means overeating and simply filling your body with whatever you want. This can lead to feeling fatigued, sluggish, and nauseous. None of those feelings are the type that you want to feel on race day, especially because of food.

Other runners mistake starch and carbs for fiber. Many starchy foods have high fiber as well. That means you'll want to skip the foods that have whole wheat and opt for foods that stay in your system longer. While the fiber in a normal diet isn't bad, fiber is notorious for cleansing the body. You certainly do not want to put stress on your gastrointestinal system right before a race. Scrambling to find the bathroom or, worse, coming down with stomach cramps is a quick way to ruin your race day experience.

Ideal starches to eat usually utilize white flour or oats. Potatoes are excellent carbohydrates to pair with proteins and vegetables. Of course, pasta is a norm for carb loading. Breakfast can also be used to build up your glycogen stores by eating oatmeal and pancakes. These are only a few examples of various starches you can use to effectively carb load.

Race Day

It's important to note that you should not be doing anything new on the day of your race. This is considered one of the golden rules of marathon racing. Ultra Marathons are no different. In addition, make sure to have your meals, snacks, gels, drinks, and any other nutrition-related needs set up and ready for the race well beforehand. Your goal is to keep your energy high today and stay prepared.

Your carb intake will need to be about every hour, so learn how much your body needs by practicing taking those carbs beforehand. In place of eating and digesting your carbs, you can also drink them, which may help with any sensations of nausea or feeling 'heavy'.

To avoid that heavy sensation, you may want to eat your last meal around 2-3 hours before your race to give yourself enough time to digest your food. But you'll also need that energy during the race itself. Your body is going to be burning through the glycogen stores quickly, and eventually, you'll experience what people call "hitting the wall, or bonking." Eating enough carbs will help keep that from happening.

During your run, you'll need to eat foods that are easy to digest. You may also want to consider both liquid and solid foods for longer runs. Make sure to practice eating while doing longer runs, well before the actual race, so your body knows how to adjust. Also, practice which kinds of foods work best with your body and provide the most nourishment well before the race, so you know what to bring with you on race day. Experiment with gels, fruit, liquid food, and simple solid foods like peanut butter and jelly sandwiches and banana toast.

HYDRATION

Most experts acknowledge that you can go 30-40 days without food, but only 3 days without water. That goes twice as much for Ultra Marathon runners. You need to keep your body hydrated, which means keeping track of your water intake. We need water to survive, and as a runner, we deplete our water stores very fast during a race. Fortunately, carb-loading also helps maintain hydration since water molecules are often stored with glycogen.

Staying hydrated is a lot harder during the race than you may think. Sometimes you may not feel dehydrated, or you might overestimate just how much water you need to take in. Finding a healthy balance is just as important to staying hydrated as the actual process of drinking water.

Water Tracking

To keep track of how much water you're drinking, you will require a combination of intentional research, body awareness, and a general understanding of your needs. **Dehydration** can cause headaches, dizziness, increased heart rate, and in severe cases, you may even stop sweating, meaning your body is no longer able to cool itself. Not only are these damaging conditions for a runner, but these can also lead to severe health problems and should not be ignored.

Taking regular drinks is important. Different experts have varying opinions about how much and how often you should drink water during your race. Most agree that you should be taking small sips more regularly rather than guzzling a gallon of water at one point during the race. Running with water sloshing around in your belly can cause discomfort and even make you feel sluggish.

Some runners swear by **drinking to thirst,** meaning that you only drink when you feel thirsty. In contrast, others say that you should drink at regular intervals no matter how thirsty you feel. This choice will be based on you and how your body feels. Every person is different; however, understanding the tools to know what works best for you will be helpful in making this decision.

The purpose of drinking to thirst is to take into consideration that everybody is different, and therefore some people may require more or less water at different rates than other people. By drinking to thirst, you allow your body to dictate its needs and provide them accordingly. You also don't have to risk over-drinking when drinking to thirst because your body will let you know when it's time.

On the other hand, planned or programmed drinking helps to prevent dehydration and overdrinking because it assesses your water intake as well as how much water you lose during the race and accommodates for that by planning regular drinking intervals. It's important to note that even if you have aid stations during your race, this method will often require you to carry liquid in some form during the actual event. This method will also use a **sweat test** to determine how much water you are losing during a race and, thus, how much water you need to continue to ingest while your body is at work.

The Sweat Test

While a sweat test is a valuable measurement of how much water you lose during a race as well as your sodium content, it is not a precise calculation that will give you the perfect number. You will still need to tailor your practice based on your own personal needs. A standard sweat test can help provide you with a general idea of how much sweat you use up and how much water you should ingest to offset that.

The sweat test itself is rather simple. Before you go for a run, weigh yourself naked. Then, for one hour, run as you normally would during your race, drinking as is natural. During this time, keep track of how much you are drinking and, if you are eating, a general idea of how much water you are getting from the food you ingest. After you finish your run, dry yourself off and weigh yourself naked again.

Now here comes the math. Take your pre-run weight and subtract the weight post-run from it. Now add the amount of water you used up on your run as well as any other liquids you were able to document consuming. This number is your total fluid lost per hour. You can divide this number however you want to determine incremental drinking planning. For example, you can divide it by four to determine how much you should drink every 15 minutes. Or by two to determine how much you should drink every 30 minutes. However you use it, you now have the information to come up with an efficient drinking plan.

Keep in mind that this method only measures your water loss for that particular moment in time. It does not take into account any other body functions that may be happening on a different day, environmental climate or conditions, terrain variations, etc. Therefore, many experts recommend that you do multiple tests to account for any variations that may not have been present during your initial sweat test.

Our Friend Sodium

Drinking a lot of water is not the only thing you need in order to be properly hydrated. In fact, drinking water without increasing your salt and sodium intake will do more harm to your body than good. There is a general myth around ingesting too much sodium. Many people think that it's bad to ingest too much sodium, when in fact, it is more harmful for you to have too little. As with anything, moderation is best. After all, no one wants to suffer from hypertension because of a high sodium diet. But without sodium, we're also unable to regulate our bodies' fluid levels. Sometimes because of low sodium levels, we may not even notice that we are thirsty, which can lead to low water intake and dehydration. This can cause a lot of damage. So during the race, you'll need to figure out how you're not just going to drink water but also get electrolytes and sodium.

There's a lot of debate about how much salt you should be ingesting during a run. And, just like hydration, there is no one answer. Your decision will probably be based on your running conditions as well as your own body. For many people, just eating something salty to recover after their race is enough. But for those like us who are training for an Ultra Marathon, we will need to ingest salt during the run. This means ingesting sports drinks that have electrolytes and other minerals as well as snacking on pretzels and potato chips provided at different aid stations. Salt tablets are not completely necessary but do provide an easy way to get a lot of salt in a short amount of time and should be considered as an alternative source.

You should also be aware of your body craving something salty. That can serve as an indicator that your balance is off and you need something to help regulate it. You can tell when you may need more salt by looking at the salt content on your skin. If you're noticing a lot of salt from sweat sticking to your skin, it's important for you to replenish that salt.

While there are many great foods that provide sodium for runners, it's important to choose foods that can help you complete your run in a healthy way. Eating a cheeseburger during a run is just not practical. However, some healthier and more reasonable options for replenishing your salt intake include salted almonds, pretzels, black olives, and many other snack foods that won't make you feel weighed down or cause you to feel sluggish.

RECOVERY AND SELF-CARE

One of the most important and overlooked steps in training your body is to recover properly. Your body deserves it. There are many different ways to recover and various methods for helping your body return to equilibrium. Recovery allows you to heal and regenerate the energy needed to perform at your best. Ironically, recovery and rest are also necessary for your body to become stronger. You can do all the running you want, but if you don't allow your body to heal your muscles and acclimate to the stress put on your system, you won't feel a marked improvement.

Recovery is actually the second part of the equation. Taking care of yourself upfront can help decrease the amount of time that you need for recovery. This means treating your body right and recognizing that it's putting in a lot of work. Your body deserves to rest, relax, and have fun. Good **self-care** means taking days off and playing a different sport or another new activity. It also means treating your limbs with care and consideration. This includes taping them up if needed, getting the right gear, regularly checking your joints and muscles to see if there are any problems, and pampering yourself every once in a while at a spa or sauna.

Methods for Recovery

There are many methods for recovering from training. One popular method involves taking an **ice bath**. As with most things, there can be controversy about the effectiveness of a good old-fashioned ice bath. Many people find that ice baths help to decrease inflammation and provide rest for tired muscles and joints. However, other specialists argue that this inflammation and adjustment period is important and decreasing inflammation actually causes more damage because the body is not allowed to heal and adjust naturally.

Maybe one of the best ways to adjust to taking an ice bath is to incorporate it into your training in such a way that it is an asset rather than a deficit. This means that you should use ice baths only when you need to recover your body from a swollen and beat-up condition. Ice baths should not be a regular thing for your body. However, when used in tandem with training and planned out beforehand, they can be a great way to refresh your legs and get relief for your body. There are even reports that claim ice baths can help you sleep better by lowering your core temperature.

To use ice baths effectively, plan on only spending a maximum of 15 minutes in the bath itself. The bath temperature should not go below 50 degrees F. That means you should not be sitting around in Arctic water. Take your time and enter the tub gradually. Don't shock your system. Only your legs and hips should be submerged in the water since they are the muscle groups you've been using the most. You should still wear clothing in order to protect your skin. Once the time is up, get out of the bath and immediately towel dry and warm up.

Eating is another essential step for recovery. Your body needs food in order to heal properly. For recovery, eating plenty of protein and foods high in vitamins and minerals gives your body the building blocks needed to patch itself together again. Carbohydrates, fats, and proteins are all involved in the body's natural recovery process. They all have important roles to play. When we exercise, we break down the protein in muscles. So we have to ingest protein in order to help build those muscles back. We also burn carbohydrates for energy and fuel. When you exercise, you've used up your stores of glycogen, and you need to replace those so that you have the energy needed for normal body functions. Fats have a more roundabout use. They are great for helping the body absorb vitamins and nutrients. Particularly those that are fat-soluble. So, while not as popular as carbohydrates or proteins, some fats are still necessary for the body to get what it needs to heal and rebuild.

Another method for taking care of your body is learning to roll out your muscles. Doing so can improve your circulation, which helps your muscles heal and adapt. It also helps to relieve the tightness you may experience from time to time around your joints and within your muscles. Rolling out your muscles with a foam roller can help you get back to training a lot faster.

This is also great for people who struggle with adequate stretching. If you know that you short-change yourself when you stretch, foam rolling can help offset some of the damage that can be missed because of inadequate stretching. Rolling out after training also helps to increase your range of motion which means that you can make better strides and utilize your body more efficiently to maintain good form and operate at your best. When foam rolling, be careful not to fall into some of the normal traps. Don't beat up your body with a foam roller—meaning don't foam roll too aggressively. Also, don't roll in only one direction. Make sure to massage your body muscles in multiple different directions to increase maximum circulation. Take time to roll slowly and intentionally across various muscle groups.

Stretching and massages both work wonders for increasing the range of motion as well as improving circulation for efficient muscle use and healing. Stretching during recovery keeps the body from knotting up and tightening the muscles. Proper stretching can keep those muscles from shortening and squeeze out natural lactic acid build-up. Stiffness and soreness are more likely to occur and remain without regular stretching after exercise. Massaging is another way that you can increase circulation and help your recovery process. Massaging is even more effective after a tough workout and if you know that you have an easy run planned the next day. Waiting at least 24 hours before strenuous exercise allows your body to repair itself and respond to massage treatment.

Rest Days

"The most important day in any running program is rest. Rest days are as important as training days. They give your muscles time to recover so you can run again. Actually, your muscles will build in strength as you rest." –Hal Higdon.

Your rest days are more important than long-run days. The rest days are where your body heals and strengthens itself. Your body requires days with no strain or strenuous activity in order to adapt to the intense pressure you have exposed it to recently. Every time you run, you break your body down in very small ways. Rest days give you the opportunity to build it back up.

This doesn't just go for your physical body; however, your mind needs the chance to recuperate as well. Doing the same thing over and over can be exhausting, and every time you run—especially if you are pushing yourself to your limits—you are putting strain on your mind. This, over a long period of time, can lead to burnout. Just like your physical body needs a rest, your mind needs a rest as well. This helps you stay motivated and focused on your training.

If you're wondering whether or not you need to have more rest days, take time to check in with yourself.

Does running feel like a chore lately rather than a fun activity? Does your body feel overwhelmed, and are you feeling more sore and unstable than usual? How is your motivation? Considering how your body and mind feel can give you a clue as to the current state of your being overall. Your mind and body come together to create one efficient running machine.

You may be wondering what you can do on your rest days if you're not allowed to work out or exercise. That part is easy. Whatever makes you feel good. For some people, they'll still move their body but will do low impact or very different exercises. Some people choose to do a very light swim, other people do some simple yoga moves that are designed to relieve stress, and others do casual cycling. If you know that your body needs even more rest and probably shouldn't move a whole lot, there is nothing wrong with sitting down with a good book or even playing computer games and allowing your mind to rest and wander to places other than the race coming up. And, of course, nothing beats a day of sleeping in and allowing a few more hours of shut-eye. Not only do you allow your body to heal and regenerate, but you also help improve your own mood and cognitive abilities in the process.

FOUR KEY ELEMENTS IN ANY ULTRA PROGRAM | 61

Taking Care of Your Joints

One of the most common questions that people ask about running is whether or not it's bad on your knees. Let's go ahead and address this issue right now. Researchers have shown that running is only bad on your knees if you have poor form or if you are increasing your training too quickly. Allowing yourself time to acclimate to your training and increasing it incrementally instead of trying to go well beyond your limits too quickly can help preserve bone and joint strength. Eating enough healthy food and taking supplements can help not only increase the rate of healing as you break down muscle and tissue but can also help improve the health and integrity of your bones.

This doesn't even take into account hydration which helps to lubricate your joints and keep the **synovial fluid** (the thick liquid between your joints) healthy.

It does deserve to be stated, however, that just because you take care of yourself doesn't mean you are exempt from knee pain or injury. Running can be hard on your knees, especially if you ignore some basic principles. For one thing, make sure you have the right kind of shoes. Knowing if you have an arch, how much support you need, and what best complements your running stride can influence the type of shoe that you should use for running.

This is especially important if you find yourself running long distances, which you will in an Ultra Marathon. A great decision by any regular runner or person who is training for a race is to find the shoe that works best for them. Ideally, you should go to a running store and have them help you. Many stores will even have you run on a treadmill and measure your gait, weight, and other factors to determine what shoe best complements your running style.

Also, be aware of the terrain that you're running on. If you are regularly running on hard, unyielding terrain like cement or concrete, then your knees and legs will be receiving the brunt of the force that you exert on that surface. But if you take time to run on softer surfaces like grass or wood, which have a little more give to them, you may find that you're able to get some good exercise in while giving your knees and bones a rest.

Knee pain can be debilitating and dangerous. If you find that you have persistent knee pain and that it impacts either your ability to run altogether or your comfort with running, take a couple of days to rest, ice your knee, and allow yourself to heal. If the pain persists or gets worse, you may need to speak with a professional to determine if there are any underlying problems. Conditions like bursitis and patellar tendinitis can cause a lot of the pain you may feel in your knee and may require a professional to take a look at in order to remedy the problem.

No matter what, the best course of action to make sure that you are taking care of your joints and bones is to run at a pace that is suitable for you. Always allow yourself time to warm up and stretch before running. Make sure that you're wearing the appropriate shoes and that you are well supported, and don't overtrain. If you find that you're experiencing pain during your running, it's time to take an extended break-even if you don't want to.

3

TIME TO GEAR UP!

"There's no such thing as bad weather, only unsuitable clothing." Alfred Wainwright made this statement in his *Coast to Coast* guidebook. Since then, the saying has appeared in commercials, ads, and many other mediums—usually relating to clothing. And why not? It may be a little facetious, but there is a large degree of truth to it.

Humans have become one of the dominant species on the planet due to our ability to reason and our ability to create and utilize tools and technology. We may not be able to run as fast as a cheetah or swim as long as a dolphin. We may not have the strength of an elephant or the reaction time of a snake, but we can circumvent all of those deficits by using our wits and our tools. Your gear is essential to your success on the race course. Even if you choose to be a minimalist and take only the bare basics, you still need tools. Your gear helps prepare you for the unknown. It gives you the edge that you need to push through situations that would otherwise be impossible.

That's not to say that people are unable to run races without gear. In fact, there are many runners who are purists and choose to run only with the clothes on their backs. But this is incredibly difficult, especially when running an Ultra Marathon. This also requires extra training because you're going to have to know how to react to inopportune situations quickly and efficiently. Your body will also need to know how to endure discomfort for long periods. This is not the recommended way to approach races, nor is it an enjoyable way to do so. The people who choose to run extra long races like Ultra Marathons this way are experts and have honed their craft to the point where they are able to do this and do it safely.

For the rest of us, we will need the correct gear and tools at our disposal to accomplish our goals. When you step out of the house to run your race, you need to ask yourself if you are properly prepared. This doesn't just apply to weather but to conditions and circumstances that may arise. Understanding your equipment and knowing what to bring is just as important for your Ultra Marathon success as training appropriately.

TEST EVERYTHING

No matter what, **you have to test everything**. If you bring any kind of gear or equipment without having tested it beforehand, you are creating a risk for yourself. Whether that means you don't know how to use the equipment properly, you lose time because you are fiddling with the equipment, or you accidentally hurt yourself or another person trying to use the equipment inappropriately; you are putting yourself at risk if you don't test everything out well in advance. This includes any equipment that you may already know how to use. Let's take something as simple as the running shoe. You've been wearing shoes since you could walk. Yet, not testing your shoes out or breaking them in before the race can put you at risk for blisters and other discomforts. Take it from me; test your equipment.

You should also test different brands to see what you like and do your research on each of these brands to understand their durability, comfort, ease of use, and effectiveness. You should also know the exact brands that work for you and of those brands which are the best and lightest that you can carry in your pack. You don't want to be weighed down by overly heavy equipment. Taking time to test your running equipment by trying them out and carrying them on a run will tell you if the gear is something that may be too heavy for you to race with.

Have the right gear, test the right gear, but no matter what, make sure that you are not leaving anything behind. You must be prepared. On race day, if you don't have something, there is a good chance you will not get it unless someone is nice and gives you what you need. But don't count on it. Your gear will depend on your environment and your race distance.

RECOMMENDED GEAR

While every runner is different and everyone has their own idea of what's important and what's not important, there are some pretty common staples that everyone knows about. As we go through this next section, we will explore some of the most common and recommended equipment runners should consider when doing Ultra Marathons. Some of these are not absolutes, and others are not optional in any way. As previously stated, no matter what gear you choose, make sure to test your equipment before race day.

Clothing

You have to wear clothes when racing not just because of the legal implications but for comfort and protection. **Running shoes** are the top most important gear that you will need to run a race. Do not go cheap on shoes. Your feet are carrying you everywhere in this race. They will be putting in the most work and are your most valuable asset. They deserve to have the best gear.

When selecting the right shoe, the first thing you need to consider is whether you will be using a trail or a road shoe. This will depend entirely on your race. Your road running shoe is designed to cope with the straightforward, high-impact, hard trails. They usually have soles that are designed to keep up with the high levels of friction between the asphalt and concrete and the rubber soles of your shoe. On the other hand, trail shoes have softer, rubber outer soles, which are useful for helping with grip and enduring the steep inclines and uneven terrain of off-road trails. Whichever shoe you decide to use, make sure that it is suited for the terrain that you'll be running in. If you'll be running on desert or beach sand, rock, or steep hills, you need the right shoe for that terrain.

A good shoe is lightly worn but not brand new. The soles and treads should be intact and sturdy; however, the inside of the shoe should feel like a well-oiled glove, gripping your foot exactly as your foot is designed. The shoe should feel secure and, most of all, comfortable. Take time to visit a running store to have your foot measured so that you know how to select your shoes or get one that is customized for your foot.

Along with your shoes, you must get socks that work for you. Again, take care of your feet. They are your most important asset. Know which socks are best for your racing environment. In the summer, you want socks that are tough but will also keep you cool and minimize blisters. Often these socks will be made of wool, bamboo, modal, polyester, or nylon. These materials have great wicking power and will keep your feet from becoming too sticky and wet. On the flip side, in order to keep your feet warm while running, you definitely need to keep moisture from getting to them. Sweat is how we cool down. So if your feet are getting wet, you can expect them to get cold. Usually, padded running socks will help to trap heat inside your shoe. You'll also want to look into wool or acrylic socks to keep moisture at bay.

You should also consider **compression socks**. These help to increase circulation and get more blood to your muscle tissues. The more blood gets to your muscle tissues, the more oxygen gets to your muscle tissues.

You need oxygen in your muscles to create energy. You also need oxygen to heal. Increasing blood circulation means that not only are you able to produce more energy, but you are not burning out your muscle fibers as fast. As you're running, your legs may swell up. That's just the name of the game. But compression socks can help reduce the swelling by increasing circulation.

Your upper body is just as important as your lower body. If you are feeling hot or cold in your upper body, eventually, that cold will diffuse to your other limbs and impact your running ability. Your shirt should be suitable for the temperature that you will be running in. Everyone has different thresholds for temperature tolerance. Try running in various temperatures to figure out what yours is. Whether you choose a **short sleeve or long sleeve shirt**, the outfit should be **wicking,** meaning that it does not hold onto moisture. You should also make sure that it doesn't chafe because you'll be making repetitive motions over and over throughout this race, and getting a rash is easy and uncomfortable. You'll also want to make sure that you get good sun protection. Getting a sunburn while running only adds to discomfort, which can be very demoralizing and even painful. Protect your skin.

Along the same lines, you should be prepared with a **lightweight wind or rain jacket**. This does not have to be thick or sturdy. In fact, it's better if it can be something that is easily folded up. The purpose of this jacket is to prepare for any surprising weather. High winds or inclement rain can throw off your body temperature and quickly make you uncomfortable.

I also highly recommend that you get a **racing vest**. They allow you to not only have an extra layer of protection but carry water and food in a simple and convenient way. If you are unfamiliar with a racing vest, it looks a lot like a vest that fits close to your body. Often they look similar to hydration backpacks, but they don't take up as much space, and they have more pockets for storage. They may not look like it, but they can store a lot of small items while taking up minimal space. They're usually lightweight and secure. Make sure that you find a vest that you like, which fits, and most of all, doesn't chafe as you run. Hydration vests can be used to carry everything and act as a *Camelbak*.

Running shorts or sweatpants should also be selected with care. Chafing is one of the biggest problems that runners have with their lower body wear. Shorts and sweatpants that do not chafe and are also wicking are the most comfortable. In most cases, you'll be using running shorts. No matter how cold it gets, your legs are usually one of the warmest parts of your body during your race, so you won't need anything longer than shorts. But in situations of poor weather, you may need to get pants that are more protective. Running shorts should also allow for a full range of motion and not be restricting in any way. Some shorts even provide a little extra support for those people who choose to do without underwear because they feel it increases their racing performance.

Beanies, hats, and gloves are usually unneeded unless you are running in cooler temperatures. Remember that your body heat will rise as you exert energy running. So you may not need this gear throughout the entire race. However, it's suitable if you know that you will be running in a colder climate or in the coolness of the evening and night. In many cases, even if you'll be running during the day, it's good to have a hat in order to protect your head from the sun.

Gaiters for your legs and **arm warmers** for your arms are purely optional. But they do provide some added support. Oftentimes, runners will forgo a long sleeve shirt in favor of a short sleeve shirt with arm warmers or shorts with leg warmers instead of sweatpants. Gaiters can help keep your legs warm, but they're also typically used to keep dirt and debris out of your shoes. Nobody likes having to stop in the middle of a race to dig a small twig or pebble out of their shoe. Gaiters come in several different sizes depending on need.

Health and Wellness

The gear you carry for your health is just as important as the gear you carry on your body. If you fail to bring any health or wellness items, you may find yourself in an emergency situation without any means to remedy it. Even if you don't use any of these items, you should have them with you just in case.

Foot powder may seem like an odd health item to bring along, but the truth is that you will most likely have some moisture build-up in your shoes if you're running for a long period of time. Hopefully, you have selected the right socks, so you don't run into that problem. But if you do, applying some foot powder is a quick way to keep blisters from forming and perspiration from collecting. The sad reality is that you will most likely lose toenails at some point. However, by adding foot powder, keeping your toenails short, and with certain kinds of socks, particularly socks with individual toe holes, you can almost eliminate the chances you will have of losing them.

Chafing creams like nut butter are another wellness item that you may not think about. Whether you are male or female, there will be times that you will experience chafing. It's very common. Usually, you'll notice because you will start to develop an itching or stinging sensation somewhere on your body. Usually, it's a combination of moisture and friction that causes that sensation to happen over time. This rubbing back-and-forth can eventually wear away skin cells and irritate your sensitive epidermis. This is how people develop rashes. Chafing cream can help decrease the friction between your legs, groin, underarms, chest, and just about anywhere else. Extended races are difficult enough without the discomfort and sticky feeling of your clothes and skin running up against each other. There are also chafing powders, but these are usually used best by applying them over a cream. That way, the powder absorbs moisture, and the cream provides support against irritation and friction.

Sunscreen is another cream that you can use to protect your skin, especially on these longer races. The last thing you want is to forget sunscreen and be fried during the race and even more miserable after. Even if you are running on an overcast day, UV rays can still get through the atmosphere and clouds and damage your skin. Because of the large amount of time that runners spend outside, you should definitely apply sunscreen. Having a small bottle of sunscreen that you can carry with you and apply or reapply as necessary can save you a lot of pain. UV light eventually denatures a lot of the elements in sunscreen over time, and you'll be sweating that protection off as well. Bringing extra sunscreen means that you'll be able to reapply it and keep your skin safe for the duration of your race.

Drop bags are pretty unique to the longer race world. Not all races have them but be prepared with them if yours don't. They are premade bags you can have ready for you at certain checkpoints. Make sure that your bag has socks, foot care, fuel, and/or drinks if needed. This is your health and wellness on the go.

A **first aid kit** is a smart choice of equipment. You never know what will happen. While there are many things that you can carry in a first aid kit, some of the most important items you can bring are blister and wound care. It does not matter how many times you have been running; you are always at risk for blisters. You can prepare and prepare as much as you want, but the little buggers often seem to rise up out of nowhere.

Wound care is also important. You are outside, in the elements, and running at a higher speed than you normally would. If you trip and fall and scrape yourself, you want to be able to react quickly and efficiently. Coincidentally, first aid is also helpful if you get stung by a bee or brush past poison ivy or any other number of natural irritations. While some situations may require further medical attention, a wisely used first aid kit can help provide a temporary solution. Along those lines, bringing along rock tape or athletic tape can help you if you stepped wrong and happened to twist your ankle or if one of your joints is feeling unstable or unsupported. A couple of wraps of tape can be just what you need in order to finish out a race.

Finally, don't ignore the importance of carrying some **toilet paper and wipes**, especially for races where you are running for multiple hours on end. You will need to use the bathroom at some point. Most likely multiple points. Having toilet paper and wipes can help you quickly handle your business, clean yourself off, and get back to the race without losing any time trying to figure out alternate solutions.

Accessories

Accessories are all of the little pieces of equipment that make your life easier. These may be items or articles of clothing. They also tend to be the ones that get forgotten the most. While many of these are optional, I still recommend them if you want to have a comfortable race.

A **water bottle** is number one on this list. It should be obvious why. You need a way to regularly hydrate and replenish the fluids that you are losing through sweat. Carrying a heavy water bottle does not make any sense.

You need a water bottle that is lightweight and easy to store. Flasks tend to fit in running vests pretty easily. They're lightweight and great for supplying hydration as you go.

Watches are another accessory that can be insanely helpful on a run. Different runners may use a watch to measure their heart rate and get an idea of how high their current intensity is. It can also be helpful to wear a smartwatch for the GPS and to know your pace and distance traveled. However, there are many runners who do not like wearing smartwatches because they don't want to be a slave to looking at the mileage. This can make the distance and time pass much slower and distract their focus from the race.

Music, while not necessary, is a great way to break up the monotony. For some people, it provides motivation and inspiration. For others, it helps calm them down and keeps them running at a steady tempo. They usually match the beats stride for stride. Music can also be distracting, however, and take away from the focus of the race. So it's entirely up to the individual to determine whether music will be a helpful accessory or not.

Trekking poles are completely optional, and most likely, you may not need them. But for many people, they are extremely helpful for races with elevation changes or simple hills. The poles relieve stress on the legs and help to propel the user forward.

Most races go into the night and may require **head-lamps**. Ideally, you should carry two of these, and you should've tested them beforehand to make sure they work and you know how to use them. This accessory will illuminate your path at night. It's dangerous to go running without that light. The last thing you want to do is run in the dark on a trail. Keep these on you, ideally in a running vest.

For longer races or races spanning a wide area, especially if you're in the wilderness, it is helpful to carry a **GPS** or **cell phone**. Many people typically have their GPS on a smartwatch or their phone. Even if you choose not to have a GPS, you should still bring your phone for emergencies. A waterproof map can also be helpful if you are running a race in which it could be possible for you to get lost.

Although it may not be as important *during* the race, you'll want to consider getting a **space blanket** for *after* the race. Space blankets were originally a military invention. They were large foil sheets that reflected the heat of soldiers back to them. This helps keep them warm during cold nights. While Ultra marathon runners are not going to war, they are still pushing their bodies to the limit.

During the race, runners generate a lot of heat because of their constant muscle movement. In response to that heat, the body does what it does best and begins to regulate the internal body temperature by sweating. The released moisture helps to cool down the body as the runner continues throughout the race. This mechanism is fantastic for runners during the race. But after the race, it can actually become dangerous. If it's cool outside and the runner has completed their race, they are no longer moving, and their body temperature is rapidly dropping. As the temperature drops, they become at risk for hypothermia. A simple space blanket can help runners recapture some of that heat so their health doesn't take a turn for the worse.

Sunglasses may seem trivial and maybe even gaudy, but they're actually a very important safety item. A good pair of sunglasses is a must for anyone who is going to be running for a long period of time. This accessory can protect your eyes from sun, dust, wind, rain, and other potentially damaging irritants. The last thing you want to do is end up squinting for hours on end as you try to pick your way down the path. If you are running in a region with a lot of insects, they also protect your eyes from accidental collisions with your buggy neighbors.

4

YOUR LOYAL CREW

Alone, we can do little; together, we can do so much.

— HELLEN KELLER

Crewing an Ultra Marathon is a significant undertaking. Crew members provide the primary support and foundation for a runner. If you have never crewed before, it's a good idea to get some crew experience before you run your first Ultra Marathon. In fact, crewing a marathon runner can be a great way to get a feel for the length and intensity of this new challenge. Not only do you get to feel the length of the day and see the condition of the runners firsthand, but you get to learn from their mistakes and their successes. Crewing for another person gives you an up-close and personal experience that you could not have in any other way by just watching.

Crewing has to do with helping a runner finish the race through support and aid at designated crew stations. This is an important task because a runner who may be on their last leg needs someone in their corner who is giving them encouraging words, food, and helping them with any other challenges they may have encountered. This slight boost can be the difference between a runner completing a race or giving up halfway through.

Choosing your crew actually comes down to who you are as a runner. This is why, when selecting your race day crew, you want to pick people that you trust. Keep logistics in mind when you think about who in your social circles may make a good crew member. Who is going to be available for race day? How far are they willing to travel? They should be organized, reliable, and actually know you as a person. They'll need to understand your racing weaknesses, the food you're able to eat, what makes you sick, what you need at various points, and your general disposition. (That may not seem important, but when you've been running for 80 miles and get cross with someone, it's easier if they already understand that you're not usually that way).

Picking this crew carefully is crucial because they will need to be self-motivated.

Often your crew will have only five minutes or less to work on you each time they see you. They'll need to be prepared with food, drinks, new socks, shoes, clothes, and any other attire that may be required. They need to be able to bandage you up if you were injured or if you have chafing and blisters. This means that they'll have to make sure to have a place for you to sit and relax while they work on you. They would also need to brush up on their basic first aid skills.

This crew will need to be able to plan for the unexpected. If they have already marked out that you will need water at a specific location but find that you are dehydrated well before then, they should have extra water bottles ready so that you can get replenished quickly. If you get injured on the way to the next checkpoint, they should be prepared to provide basic first aid and assist you with finding extra help if needed.

THE RACE DAY CREW

This is your master team. The team is made up of a set of crew members and typically one crew leader. Make sure to check with your race to make sure that they allow crews. Not all races do. If the race doesn't allow crews, that's okay; just make sure that you have an excellent support team instead.

Naturally, many people may choose those that they are closest to, like family members. They're often some of the first choices to be part of the race crew. That makes sense. It's a big event in your life, so you want people who have shown support for you in the past to be part of it.

With a bit of creativity, there is likely something that everyone can do during the race, even if it's not one of the leading roles. For example, parents or grandparents may be great at taking pictures - even though they may not know what or where to do anything else. Or, you can find someone who is able to provide long-distance support by babysitting children or pets so that you won't have any distractions or concerns. Your mind will need to be as focused as possible, and if, for example, you are concerned about one of your kids having a meltdown, that may throw you off.

If one of your family members has been in a crew before and can dedicate the time, they might be a prime candidate for your team. However, keep in mind that being in the crew can get busy and demanding. If your family member simply wants to be in the moment, it may be better for them to serve as general support rather than as a member of the crew.

So let's say you've chosen your crew. You should plan to meet about 2-5 days before the race just to get an idea of expectations and play out different scenarios. This is really for the crew to have an idea as to how to respond to the runner. For example, when the runner says that they cannot eat at the moment they should be eating, what should the crew do or say? Similarly, if the runner says their Achilles tendon is on fire and they can't go on, what are some remedies the crew should suggest?

Perhaps the most important question is to ask the runner how the crew should know when it is truly time to call it quits. This isn't something runners like to talk about because the idea of not finishing a race you've spent months of hard work preparing for is a terrible feeling. But the reality is that in any Ultra Marathon, there will be runners who, for one reason or another, won't make it to the finish line. Understanding what the point of no return looks like is important because it also will dictate how much the crew should push you and when they should tell you to stop.

If you want to take your race crew to the next level, you could also assign specific roles to other members, just like you did with the crew leader. Two other positions that Ultra Marathon participants will sometimes select are a logistics manager and a communicator.

The logistics manager is the person who will coordinate things like distance to the checkpoint, directions, the best mode of transportation there, along with things like parking considerations. They would also be keeping track of what may be needed at each point, such as fuel and hydration. They should have an in-depth understanding of the race guide and know how to navigate specific rules like the number of people allowed in the tent at each checkpoint. If you know someone who likes planning and spreadsheets, they just might be your person for this role.

The communicator is the person who, as you might guess, communicates between the runner, other crew members, and race personnel. For example, say you decide that you will want a different pair of shoes at a certain time or need to see a medic, the communicator can be the one to facilitate that information.

Note that even with the crew assignments, the crew leader is still in charge of the whole operation. But sometimes, it helps to assign more roles to other members of the team so that responsibilities are better delegated and covered.

Crew Leader

Your crew leader is your main person. They are the one who takes charge and helps direct everyone else to know what to do. Having five people trying to do the same thing at once with no order gets bad and frustrating.

The crew leader is in charge of splitting the crew among the different aid stations or organizing them so that they can make sure to be at each waypoint at the correct time. They are also in charge of making sure that everyone knows where they should be and when. While the entire crew should be educated on the race, the crew leader is the main one to carry out the wishes of the runner. They are usually involved in making lists and studying the maps. They make sure to distribute the food and drinks that the runner will need at each waypoint. Every single detail is important, and it's up to the crew leader and the runner to determine precisely how and when everything should be presented.

The crew leader will also be the person who doles out responsibilities to the crew at each aid station. This means knowing which aid stations are providing food, and medical attention, providing the runner information on the next portion of the race, or just doing a time check.

The crew leader will also be providing support to the rest of the crew. They'll be in charge of making sure that everyone else is staying hydrated, rested, and well-fed. A crew is only able to provide optimal support to the runner if they are taking care of themselves as well. It can be easy to get wrapped up in planning and the excitement of the race and forget to care for yourself. The crew leader is in charge of making sure that the crew is staying healthy (or designating someone to be in charge of that).

Crew leaders should also be the most familiar with the runner and ready to be on call at any given moment. While it's nice if they can be at every aid station along the way, oftentimes, it can be impractical. However, they should make sure to be aware of everything going on and be ready to make split-second decisions if necessary.

When considering who would make a good crew leader, look at someone who is confident and able to make swift decisions. They should be able to explain clearly what needs to happen and be able to point others in the right direction. Consider the personalities of the people around you. Who seems to be a natural leader? Who would be passionate about your success in this race?

Pacers

Pacers are not always allowed in races. So, it's important to know the rules about pacers well before you start your race. These are people you choose to run with you at specific points of the race to help you keep going and stay motivated. Make sure you understand the race rules regarding pacers because some pacers will need to have a racers bib or a crew ticket in order for them to join you. Some races may only allow you to have a pacer after passing a certain point in the race or accumulating enough mileage.

A pacer is important because they help you maintain a regular pace along your run. These pacers may not be in the kind of shape that you are, and they may need to trade out every so often so that they can stay fresh. Their goal is to keep you motivated and inspired to maintain your running speed. Their duties include keeping track of your pace and monitoring the clock so that you are hitting each of your milestones at the correct time and at the pre-designated moment. Pacers can help distract you from challenging moments in the race, and they can also provide emotional support and encouragement so that you can push past your limits.

The best pacers on a crew are able to simultaneously maintain the runner's ideal pace while also paying close attention to the runner themselves. They are able to pick up on cues that tell them if the runner needs someone to talk to or if they just need to run in silence. These are also details that should be discussed during the crew team meeting beforehand. Pacers are helping to set the ambiance for the runner and should know exactly what is expected of them before they end up next to the runner on the trail.

Similarly, the runner needs to be open and honest about what they need from the pacer. They should also be intentional about meeting the same pace as their pacer unless they decide otherwise beforehand. There have been many situations where an overzealous runner took off ahead of his pacer, rendering the crewmember useless. Now, if this is an expectation and outlined beforehand as a possibility, then the pacer knows that their job is to simply maintain the pace no matter what.

They may continue to maintain the pace even if the runner falls behind them and the pacer is ahead of the runner. Seeing the back of the pacer, who represents their ideal time, can be great motivation for a runner to pick up the pace and push past the wall that they may have hit. If the pacer had not communicated with the runner, however, they may have stopped and gone back to join and encourage them. Then the runner would never have experienced that pulse of motivation.

While pacers do not need to be at the same level of fitness as the runner, they should be training beforehand to meet the required distance they will be running with them. This means that pacers need to be runners in their own right. They also need to have training plans and be ready to perform on race day.

Support Team

Even if you're unable to have a crew or pacers, you'll need support before and after the race. Trying to go through the Ultra Marathon experience solo is 100 % possible and people do it all the time. However, having a few people there to encourage you as you begin and to be ready to receive you when you end can provide the energy you need to start a race and end it.

A support team is also there to help with all the things an average crew team would assist you with. The only difference is they can't be there at certain points throughout the race. Even so, at the beginning of the race, there are many little details that you don't want to have to think about when you're trying to prepare your mind for the race. Then, there will be things that you just can't think about at the end of the race when you're so exhausted that you just want to drop onto the grass and not get back up.

Your support team can help make decisions at the beginning of the race and get you organized and ready. They can also help relieve you of any concerns that you carry with you to the starting line. Even if that means they need to check to make sure that the stove is off. Every wandering and distracting thought can be the thought that separates you from completing the race and giving up in the middle. A good support team will be there at the end of the race with hydration and snacks, and maybe even a warm blanket to catch you safely.

5

THE MENTAL BATTLE

U p to this point, we've talked about how to prepare for your first marathon—where to begin, running gear, support crew, etc. Most people think the race starts when you step out onto the course and after the gun goes off. However, I would argue that those who go in with this thought process are already at a disadvantage. The first battle that takes place happens before you lace up your shoes. The first battle is the one in which you are your sole competitor. It is the battle of the mind.

This battle is a war of attrition. Throughout the course of training and even going into the race, you will have dozens of conflicting thoughts. Each thought is vying for your complete attention and submission. The thought you allow to continue and grow is going to shape your belief and perspective. It's here, at the cross-roads of decision, that runners make the choice of whether they are going to stay in the race and finish at all costs or allow space for them to quit.

I'm not talking about quitting because of an injury, a family emergency, or some other disaster beyond your control. I am speaking entirely about deciding whether or not this race is too hard for you. The majority of runners who quit in the middle of these large-scale races had already made that decision long before they began the race or felt the pain of their body's muscles being challenged.

Coming into the race with anything less than full commitment to completion is already setting yourself up for failure. When you enter this arena, you need to make a conscious decision that you will see this through. That conviction is what will carry you through the difficulties and tough trials ahead. This attitude is what sets the hobbyists apart from the athletes and competitors.

THE POWER OF THE MIND

There's a very old story about a man who worked at the railroad station. His job was to document all of the cargo on the rails the night before to make sure that they were properly accounted for. He did his job diligently checking each cargo hold one by one and carefully making note of everything that was supposed to be in each car.

One night as he checked the cargo, as usual, he stepped into one of the freezer containers for meat and produce. The latch for the door was faulty, and as he marked the freezer car as empty, he heard the door slide shut with a resounding click behind him. Immediately, panic set in. He realized that it would be over 12 hours before anyone found him the next morning.

He searched the empty container for any items or tools he could use to try to force his way out. But after fighting with the door for over an hour, he finally fell to the floor in resignation. Knowing he would eventually die as the cold set in, he took his notebook where he'd been documenting all the contents of the containers and flipped the page, pressing his pen to the paper and writing a letter to his wife. He described his love for her and then began to outline his last moments. He described the way that his skin began to grow cool to the touch, and he could feel his insides start to freeze. He talked about the way that his teeth began to chatter and how he drew himself into a ball, trying to keep himself warm. Twelve hours later, his body was discovered by railroad workers. The man lay dead in an unplugged, room temperature freezer car.

Our minds are capable of incredible things. In the case of this man, he was so certain that he was going to freeze to death that his mind made him think he was freezing even though he wasn't in reality. Our mind has the ability to play tricks on us, to run away, to create anxiety and panic-like feelings, and to stimulate our nervous system. We can either allow our minds to wander and do as they wish, or we can take control of them and use them as our greatest strength.

There will be moments when your body feels like it cannot continue, and you will need to engage the power of your mind to convince your body that it can. Our bodies are capable of much more than we think or feel that they are. But often, we can't tap into that strength unless we are intentional about how we use our minds. If you begin a race thinking entirely about how hard it is, how long the distance is, how much time it will take, or how much better-prepared everyone else is than you, you'll fail. You've already convinced yourself that you are not capable of handling this task. On the other hand, if you convince yourself that you have prepared for this, that you are capable of going the distance, and that this will be a fun and enjoyable experience for you, suddenly, your worldview has changed.

We call this perspective. Our perspective has the power to color the way that we see things, and it directly affects our attitude. Think about how many times you've come home from work and didn't feel like doing something as mundane as mowing the lawn. Even if you work at a job where you're not active all the time, and so your body itself has plenty of energy, your mindset and perspective have already told you that it has been a long day and you would rather relax than mow the lawn. While this may not be a big deal in this situation, it is a huge deal when you are trying to accomplish the significant goal of completing an Ultra Marathon. Your perspective during this marathon is essential.

TRAINING YOUR MIND

The beauty of the mind is its capacity to learn and develop. Even if our mind reacts one way, we can teach it to react differently. Sometimes that process may take a while. Other times it may seem to happen quickly. But fast or slow, our mind has the ability to be molded and shaped. We just have to be intentional about training it, just like we are with our bodies.

While you are definitely training your mind while you train your body, there is something to be said about intentionally seeking out the places where the story you tell yourself is holding you back. When you are able to find those places where your mind weakens, you can figure out how to push through to accomplish your goal. But you won't know where and how to do this unless you do some self-reflection first.

When you are training for a marathon, you have your training plan. But you also regularly evaluate yourself to determine if you are going at a good enough speed, using the proper form, and pacing yourself correctly. At every moment, you are continually evaluating and adjusting so that you can get better.

What many runners don't realize is that your mind can benefit from the same attention. After a run, take a moment to evaluate how you felt during that run. What is your mindset? Are you agitated or worried? Did you feel distracted or noisy? How is your confidence level? Did you feel like you were capable of completing this phase of training, or were you doubtful?

These questions help to begin to outline the story that you tell yourself as you are running. They serve as an introduction to evaluating your mental fortitude and conviction. Where you find negativity or doubt, those are places to dig deeper and better understand the emotion or thought behind the negativity. Doing so helps you remove another hurdle to your ultramarathon success.

Running and Mental Toughness

During the American Revolution, the British, on paper, should have won. They had the numbers. They had the money. They had the equipment. While the argument can be made that Americans had the advantage of home turf, I would argue they had something that far outweighed the British army—guts and grit. They were willing to sacrifice it all for what they believed in. They knew their why. Now, why am I telling you this? Because even the greatest athletes who have done all the preparation can lose to what some may call the underdog. Because at the end of the day, what usually separates the good from the great, isn't the extra hours in the gym; it's the mental toughness they've also worked on.

At some point during your race, you are going to be in pain. Maybe it's just the normal pain of exhaustion or the mental pain of fatigue and weariness. Whatever the case, you will feel uncomfortable, and you'll need something to pull you through. This is where mental toughness comes in.

One of the most important things you can do to increase your mental toughness is to accept that you are going to feel stressed during your run. There is going to be a strain on your body, and you're going to feel tired. Remember this, even when you are doing really well in your training, and it feels like you're not even trying anymore. Remind yourself over and over what you are doing is tough, and you have to push through it. That mantra in your mind is what will carry you through that moment when you feel the first twinge in your leg. That mindset will push you through when your lungs begin to heave and your chest begins to hurt. This is all part of the process. None of this is unexpected. You can do this because you knew it was coming.

Another way you can build your mental toughness is to develop a series of memories that prove you are capable of overcoming hard things. Think of this as a mental photo book. When you encounter something difficult, there is a psychological dialogue that begins to happen between two parts of you. The part that wants to continue and the part that wants to quit. The dialogue will go something like this:

"Wow, this is really difficult. I think it's time to give up."

"Oh, but I've worked so hard for this. I really want to keep going. Imagine what it would be like to feel the success of accomplishing this."

"No, no this isn't fun anymore. I don't like this feeling, and I want to stop. You have to keep going. Do I want to keep going?"

Once you begin to have a conversation similar to that and those thoughts begin to roll through your mind, it's time to take out your photo book. As you mentally flip through this photobook, you'll be able to draw on different occasions to prove to the brain that wants to quit that you don't need to quit. You are capable of doing this.

Maybe it's the first time you completed a marathon. The euphoria and relief after you finished. The confidence you felt that now you are capable of completing marathons. Or maybe it's the celebration after your first 50k. Sitting around the table at the restaurant with your friends and family and realizing that you aren't alone in your crazy running adventures. You can even draw on training. Think about how many times during training you questioned whether or not this was worth it. Think about the times that you sacrificed other things in favor of honing your body and pushing past your current limits. That was hard, but you did it.

This photo book defines your ability to surpass what seems impossible. And as you flip through that mental photo book, you are going to remind yourself that just like you overcome all of those other obstacles, you will overcome this one. All you have to do is keep pushing through it.

Something else you can include in your mental photo book is the images of why you chose to do this race in the first place. Again, there will come a time where your dialogue will be between the brain that wants to continue and the brain that wants to quit. That conversation may sound something like this:

"This hurts so much. Why did I choose to do this?"

"I can do this. I can press through; I know I can."

"This is so stupid. I was never meant to be able to do something like this; I should just quit."

"Oh, but I really want to continue forward."

Again, this dialogue is at a stalemate until you begin to bring in your photo book and start reflecting on all the reasons that you decided to try this Ultra Marathon. This is the moment to reflect on all the people who stood behind you and said that you could do this, that this was right up your alley.

Or, this is the time to reflect on all the people who thought it was impossible for you to accomplish this. Think about how bad you wanted to prove them wrong. Think about your desire to surpass your limits and to continue to push your body to new heights. Think about the experience overall—doing such a grandiose race, something that so few people ever do.

This is an experience that is unique, and you get to take part in it. This collection of reasons why you are doing this race will give you an extra push to finish strong.

Think about when you are stretching. There's a point when you feel like you've reached your peak. It's at that time that you should lean in a bit further because that is where the growth happens. The next time you try that stretch, you will be able to go further than you did the last time. It's painful, but over time it becomes less and less painful, and you grow in the process. Just as you spend time strengthening your muscles and stamina, it's important to spend time building your mental toughness.

Mental Preparation

There are many approaches to strengthening your mind. I believe the first place is to start outside of the gym and off the course. **Prepare your mind through meditation, visualization, understanding your why, and self-affirmation.** Depending on what your spiritual background is, the idea of meditation may feel familiar or foreign. However, in today's society, the ability to be still and refocus is much more difficult due to the many distractions around us—our screens, social media, work, family, on top of your own mental noise.

Meditation is an excellent way to quiet some of those external factors and find your center. Meditation has been studied and shown to reduce anxiety and stress, improve focus, increase pain tolerance, and even increase cardiovascular health by decreasing blood pressure and increasing oxygen capacity in the lungs. All of this sounds great, but even with meditation, it is best to start small and work your way up. Let me also put this disclaimer that the beauty of meditation is that there is no right or wrong way to do it. If it works for you and you find benefit, that's the right way for you. If you find certain styles aren't helping, it may be time to switch the routine.

Give yourself a bit of grace and know that imperfect meditation is better than none at all. Practice makes progress, not perfection. If you have never done it before, perhaps start by finding a corner in your home and spending five minutes a day simply being still. During this time, there are several things you can think about, and there are many applications for meditation. However, as far as training for a marathon, I believe this segues into the next aspect of mental preparation.

While you meditate, it can be helpful to think about why you want to run. What does it do for you? Better yet, who are you running for? Creating an emotional attachment can fuel your determination when you get on the course. Some people may decide that they run in memory of a loved one. What a beautiful way that is to honor them and perhaps give space for a healthy outlet for grief.

Some people find that running for a charity allows them to run for a reason outside of themselves, which can be a powerful motivating factor. Others run as a way to build self- empowerment. Still, others may run as a symbol for a major lifestyle change. Others find that peer pressure is a motivating factor. If you are able to find other like-minded people who go out to run, you are more likely to follow suit, especially on the days you don't feel like it. There is something motivating about not wanting to let the team down. On the other hand, many find that running brings a level of solitude that they may not have much of during the day. It can allow for space to clear your head of the thoughts of the day or your concerns. It can provide a release from stress. If stress reduction is needed, and let's be real, who couldn't use a little less stress in their life, then running may give purpose to that end. If your New Year's resolution was to get outside more, running could be an avenue to fulfill that. Getting out more in nature and taking in more fresh air could be your why. Whatever it is, you can use meditation as a way to think about what beyond your muscle will propel you forward, especially when your muscles are begging for mercy.

Next, visualize where you will be running. As much as possible, use all five senses as you visualize. Close your eyes. Imagine yourself running on your favorite trail. As you deeply inhale, you can smell the crisp air that is fragrant with blooms of spring. With each step, you hear the sound of the pavement colliding with the sole of your foot, providing a secure surface for you to push yourself forward. From a distance, you see a small clover that has poked through the pavement. It gets closer and closer until you gently glide over it so as not to disturb it. You take a sip of water and notice the salty aftertaste from the sweat above your lip. You make your way to the dreaded hill. No, not dreaded. It's just a hill, and you are going to attack it with everything you have.

Some runners find it helpful to make the difficult parts of the course a symbol. For example, you imagine you are attacking the hill just like the children supported by your charity attack chemotherapy. Visualize each part of the course. Uphill, downhill, turns, and the landmarks. Think about every moment. The beginning is when you start, and the end is when perhaps your loved ones are cheering you on as you finish. Visualize finishing and meeting your goal. All of this may sound corny, but think about it, if you can't imagine reaching your goal, it likely won't suddenly manifest itself on race day.

Lastly, during your meditation, you can affirm yourself. This is where you can start by thinking about where you started—the hours of preparation. The moments you wanted to give up but pushed through. This is when you tell yourself that you are ready for this. Not just because you're able to think it, but because you have measurable action behind it. You are a warrior. You have never been stronger than where you are right now. Every step in life up to this point has aided in your preparation. The more self-confidence you build, the more fear will fall. It's okay to tell yourself that there may be pain and that perhaps you don't like the idea of that. Be honest. But for every reason, think back to your why instead of thinking about a why not.

The other reason why meditation may be helpful is because it allows you to get to know yourself on a more intimate level. When you begin to have pain, you will start to understand whether the pain is something you can or should mentally push through or if mental toughness isn't the problem and you need to take a rest. Essentially you will start to tell the difference between good pain and bad pain. There are a few red flags to consider when trying to discern the difference. The first is, how severe is the pain? Is it bad enough to where you are having to alter your gait to compensate? Is it a four or five out of ten or higher? If so, it's definitely time to get checked.

Some other indicators include the asymmetry of the pain. This may suggest that there is a local injury versus generalized musculoskeletal pain that is expected of aerobic training. You also shouldn't be in pain for more than 24 hours. If you are in pain for longer than a day, it is a sign you probably need to cut back the amount of training and allow your body more time to rebuild. Know your physical limits before you run. I'd like to affirm that cutting back due to concerns about injury says nothing about your mental toughness. In fact, sometimes, the most challenging thing you can do is step back when all you want to do is plow forward full steam ahead.

That moment is where you find what you are made of. This is where you find yourself. On the subject of running, Kristin Armstrong said, "There is something magical about running; after a certain distance, it transcends the body. Then a bit further, it transcends the mind. A bit further yet, and what you have before you, laid bare, is the soul." She might not have realized it, but she is perfectly describing the phenomenon of **runner's high**.

Runner's high refers to the euphoric state athletes may feel after a long duration of intense workout. It is caused by the release of endorphins which have similar effects on the body as morphine, a powerful pain reliever. Additionally, a flood of neurotransmitters is released, including norepinephrine, dopamine, and serotonin. Norepinephrine helps to boost mood, focus, and energy. Dopamine helps the motivation and the reward pathway. In other words, the release of dopamine during a run is more likely to motivate you to do it again. Lastly, serotonin can help decrease anxiety, improve mood, and help with sleep. Some of the most significant benefits from running happen when you push yourself a little further than you thought you could go.

All that sounds nice, but you're perhaps thinking, but how do I get there when the pain makes me want to stop? Well, there are a few things. The first important thing is to take your mind off the pain. There is a concept called diabolic learning. Essentially it's the idea that your brain has the capacity to learn and grow. However, if cycles of suffering and pain are not broken, it will simply learn to expect and be more sensitive to pain.

On the other hand, the more one engages in enjoyable activities, the more it will learn to be happy and produce happy hormones. So when you start to have pain, don't focus solely on the pain. Think about how grateful you are to have the ability to run. Think about how beautiful your surroundings are. Or take time to notice the beauty around you. Think about your why. Think about how strong you are—how much stronger you are than the pain.

6

LET THE RACE BEGIN

Once you begin the race, that's it. There is no more training. No more preparation. The only conversations you'll be able to have with your crew will be brief and pointed. Now is the time to put everything into play. This may seem daunting. All that's left is the sense of anticipation as you wait for the starting signal.

PREPARATION IS KEY

Many people focus on the weeks leading up to the race and the day of the race itself. However, the few days leading up to the race are just as crucial in terms of preparation. Not only does the race get much more difficult. This is an ideal time to communicate with your team and let them know everything you'll need from them. Talk to your crew leader and organize the team and the flow of the race. Everyone needs to be on the same page.

Make sure all of your gear is tested and that you are comfortable with every item that you'll need. While I don't recommend making any new changes too close to the race, if something isn't working properly or an issue comes up, it is better to know beforehand rather than on race day. The same goes for food and hydration. Be cautious about changing any diet issues close to the race. Your body has become accustomed to a specific set of nutrient requirements. Straying too far from your routine may throw your body off balance and cause more upset on race day than any benefit.

If possible, try to scout the course before race day, whether in person or virtual. Learn as much as you can so you won't be caught off guard by the terrain, incline, or any helpful landmarks. You especially want to map out where each checkpoint is and what will be at each one, particularly in terms of hydration and fuel. Communicate with your team to find out which check-points you will meet them at. When packing for your first race, it may be tempting to cram as much as you can in your hydration vest. I want to emphasize that this is why it is important to study checkpoints as much as possible. This will dictate what is necessary for you to carry on the day of versus what you can count on at checkpoints.

The weather may be another factor to consider. You may want to watch the weather the week and days leading up to the day of the race. If you are looking to chase a time goal, you may want to consider changing races. However, if you are running for other reasons like conquering the race, running with friends, or for a cause, the weather may not affect you, but you may still want to be mindful of factors like humidity and temperature. Even though you will not have run the race, by the time race day comes, you should be so familiar with your own mind, body, and course that the day of the race simply feels mundane. This will allow you to reach an optimal balance of calm and focus. Lastly, just know that no matter how much you prepare, there may still be something that goes wrong. Roll with the punches. Fix one thing at a time.

Imagine that today is the day you have been preparing for—race day. The moment you wake up, you may start having thoughts and feelings ranging from excitement to nervous anticipation. It is all normal. Take a few deep breaths and if it helps, do some meditation before or while you get ready in order to calm your mind and allow you to focus better.

Have you noticed that when you are running alone, you have a heightened sense of physical awareness? Suddenly you notice that perhaps your shoe is slightly off-center or the ache in your knee. It's interesting how when the crowds are present, and there is noise, how much these things might not bother you as much. This is because when you are alone, your mind has little else to focus on other than its internal state. When you are alone, it will be easier for you to fixate on discomfort and your levels of fatigue and exhaustion. Being alone can be difficult, but it can also be a time where you can engage in positive self-talk and challenge some of the negative thoughts you may have during the race.

BEST PRACTICES

You are not the first person to do an Ultra Marathon. In fact, you are not the first person to do any length of race. Hundreds of people have gone before you and have had their own experiences, successes, and failures. One of the best things you can do as someone who is a new runner or new to Ultra Marathons is to pick the brains of all of those who came before. Ask runners for their experience and their advice. Many of them are happy to share the things that have worked for them. You don't have to take every piece of advice that they offer, but it will give you a good idea of the things you need to consider to be successful.

A wise person chooses to listen to the advice of those with more experience than them. Running is no different. There are a lot of common themes that can be found among runners and in this community. While specifics may differ from person to person, there are some general points that I believe everyone can agree on.

Slow and Steady

There is often the question of how to pace yourself during the race. Even those running marathons typically don't run the entire distance during training. On race day, it's recommended to run 1-2 minutes per mile slower than what you would during training. The most important thing is to understand your own fitness level when determining pace. Remember that your marathon race day will be a compilation of all of your training. You, as well as the other runners, are likely just trying to finish the race rather than finish first. That being said, don't be tempted to keep pace with other runners at the beginning. Some miles will be more challenging than others, and natural elements like the wind could also affect how fast you go. The key is not to let adrenaline at the start take control of the race and dictate your pace. If you are running as fast as you did during training, you are likely running too fast. Start slow, and end slower.

During the race, breathing is such an important element. Not only does it help to provide your body with adequate oxygen, but it can also give you a rhythm or a cadence for how you should run. Some people like to make a pattern where they take four breaths in through their nose and four breaths out through their mouth. They do this and think of their running pattern. If you feel like you're gasping for air or starting to feel more tired, you can always change up the breathing pattern. For example, you could modify it to take two breaths or three breaths but still keep the pattern and sync with your stride. Since it's something new, you could try doing it for 30 seconds to one minute at a time and see how it feels.

Another breathing technique you can use is called belly breathing. If you do yoga, you might be familiar with this term. For most runners, especially when you start getting tired, it's more natural to bring your shoulders into a shrug as you inhale. This isn't as optimal as belly breathing. Belly breathing is the exact opposite in which you take a deep breath and allow your belly to expand rather than contract. This will allow your lungs to expand fully. The best way to practice this is by simply lying on your back on the floor and practicing breathing in through your nose, allowing your belly to come away from the floor and exhale through your mouth, allowing your belly to sink in and help release the rest of the carbon dioxide. You can also inhale and exhale on a count similar to what was described previously.

Now, I've talked a bit about cadence as it relates to breathing. Running occurs on a rhythm. If you've played a musical instrument, you're familiar with the term cadence. When they are practicing, musicians will often use a device called a metronome. The purpose of the metronome is to keep a particular beat that allows the musician to stay on tempo. Similarly, when running, it can be helpful to have an internal or external system to help you develop a cadence and stay on your target. Contrary to what may be intuitive, having a faster cadence may help you better achieve your goals in the long run. This is because running on a slower cadence means that you are stretching out your stride and may be more prone to injury. A quicker cadence implies that you're taking shorter strides. This means less pressure on each step, which is less tiring in the long run.

Trust Your Training

In the time leading up to the race and perhaps on race day itself, you will likely run into other runners who may talk about their approach to training, nutrition, experience, etc. If this is your first race, it could be easy to become distracted or intimidated by so many different opinions. This is not the time to start trying to change your practices. This is the time to trust your own preparation.

Remember that everyone will have a different way of going about the race, but you should not be swayed, especially in the final hours. You have spent weeks not just training but getting to know yourself. You know best what works for you. You know your body. You know your strengths and weaknesses. Your training has prepared you for the race.

You may also start to feel some anxiety, wondering if you have everything that you need, if you should've prepared some more, and doubting your abilities. This is normal. In some ways, it may even be healthy. But obsessing and repeatedly playing visions of failure in your mind is not the way to achieve your goal. There's nothing wrong with checking and rechecking your preparations. But doubting yourself and undermining your training will be more damaging than helpful.

During moments where you begin to feel anxious or unsure about whether you're ready for this challenge, remind yourself of all of the things that you have done. Play through your mind every step, every mile, every conversation you've had with your support team, and all of the long hours spent planning your nutrition and becoming familiar with your fear. These seemingly small actions can help you build confidence in yourself. When you see how you have paid attention to the most minute details, you'll gain a better appreciation for the process you followed to get here.

When you take that first step, there is no place for doubt. Your mind needs to either be committed to running this race or walking away. You are ready. You have done the work. Now trust your body to follow through with the rest. Once you get into a rhythm, your training will take over. If you were allowed to have a crew team, they would be there to assist you. You have all of the gear and supplies that you'll need. The only thing left is for you to run the best race you can.

Keep the Tank Full

During the race, it is crucial to remain hydrated and adequately fueled. It's easy to simply take advantage of what is at the checkpoint. But you have several options to consider. Energy gels for runners are popular because they are an easy way to get fast carbohydrates to your body. However, some runners prefer having 'real' food like bananas, apple sauce, or dates. The most important thing is to eat what feels good for you.

Experiment a bit before race day. It can be challenging to find your rhythm when you're trying to eat and drink while running, especially for your first race. Some runners even say it's awkward. You might be tempted to skip and try to make it to the next fuel station. However, if you start feeling that temptation, avoid it. You absolutely need to keep food in your stomach so that you have the energy to continue and so your muscles get the nutrients they need.

Remember to drink water as well. If your fuel has salts or electrolytes, you might not have to use Gatorade or other sports drinks as often. However, it will be vital that you remain hydrated—especially if you are running in warmer or more humid conditions that cause you to lose fluids. You should plan to refuel every hour even if, at the moment, you don't think you need it.

It's actually best to fuel before you feel you need to. Keep in mind that if you don't take the proper time to fuel, your body won't have the nutrients it needs to endure such a harrowing ordeal. Oftentimes runners that don't properly fuel will hit a wall. They may run out of glycogen stores which is the way your body stores extra glucose. Without glycogen, you may experience muscle cramping, fatigue, and dizziness. Not only will poor fueling impact you physically, but it may impact you mentally. Your brain requires a lot of glucose in order to complete its functions—this includes focus and attention. Without fuel, it will be more challenging to remain in the present and put to practice any meditation or mind training you've done previously.

Appreciate the Solitude

Runners often overlook how alone they will be while running on the day of the race. This can be a difficult realization to have during the excitement and anxiety of race day, especially when you are in between checkpoints. Studies have shown that runners tend to run faster when faced with overt competition rather than when compared with their time trial run alone. Studies have also shown that regardless of the difficulty level of the race, when runners have to run alone, they are more likely to perceive increased exertion and have more subjective negative feelings about the race. That being said, it is important to prepare to run alone from a mental standpoint.

Even if you are in a race with lots of people, there will likely come moments where no one will be around you. That's why your motivation cannot be keeping up with other people or trying to beat the time of the other participants. Your motivation must come from within, driven by a desire to do the best that you can as a runner. During moments like these, it can be helpful to learn to appreciate solitude.

In our world, we are often bombarded with the presence of other people. Whether it be living in a house with other people, exposure to the lives of others on social media, or listening to talking heads on television. Most of us are used to having the presence of people around us. And that's OK. We were not intended to be islands. In fact, human beings are social creatures. We like connection. So in those moments during your race, when you are by yourself, you have to learn to break through that feeling of disconnection.

During these moments, find ways to enjoy that feeling of being alone rather than fearing it. Have music or a podcast ready to distract your mind and provide a simple form of entertainment. Take a moment to appreciate the scenery or nature around you. Play simple games with yourself, trying to spot different items or landmarks. Compose a song, poetry, or a story in your mind. Or think through a challenging situation that you've been facing recently and try to come up with solutions or a different way of looking at it. Plan out how you're going to celebrate your race completion. There are numerous ways to appreciate solitude during your run. Find a few techniques that work for you and practice them during your training. That way, when you get to race day, you will automatically slip into that train of thought and begin practicing your appreciation during those moments of solitude.

Be Prepared for Tough

No matter how much you prepare, there will likely be something that happens on race day that is simply out of your control. In the 2016 Rio Olympics, Abbey D'Agostino of the United States and Nikki Hamblin of New Zealand lined up with the other runners for the second 5000m heat. With anticipation, the runners approached the starting line, all ready to leave everything out on the track. Every moment of training and sacrifice had led them to this monumental moment in their running career.

The gun went off, and the runners converged down the track. Shortly after the start of the race, Hamblin and D'Agostino both took a tumble. The other runners kept going. D'Agostino was the first to rise and check on Hamblin. It appeared that she was okay and more concerned about her fellow athlete. After helping Hamblin to her feet, she then attempted to resume the race, but it wasn't until then she realized how much pain she was in. Everyone held their breath while watching her take steps gingerly, each one sending shockwaves of pain that radiated into her facial expressions. In spite of the pain, in spite of the disappointment, D'Agostino was determined to keep running to finish the race. She was the last one on the track, and yet the crowd began to roar as she finally made her way toward the finish line. In an interview following the event, she said, "it certainly wasn't the experience we thought we were going to have, but we're on an adventure to see what happens...."

Now, of course, this is a different event and setting; however, the Olympics are considered to be one of the ultimate battlegrounds for athletes—many of whom train their entire lives so that they can perform at their best. I'd imagine for either Hamblin or D'Agostino that getting caught up in the jumble of runners at the start and falling to the ground was not in their training plans. I can further imagine that D'Agostino hadn't planned to have a severe injury from the fall that not only limited her performance in the race but would require months of healing going forward.

Yet, even with the immense curve ball they were both thrown, they chose to roll with the punches and focus on something greater than themselves. I encourage you to be as prepared as you can, but when an unexpected issue arises, and from experience, I can promise they will, try to remain calm. You might get sick, roll your ankle, have storm clouds roll in, suffer heat exhaustion or dehydration, or have an injury. When a curveball comes, assess the problem. Ask yourself if this is something to work past? Assess for injury and safety—whether or not to continue. Some of this may be based on how far you have to go in the race. If possible, solve the problem and get back to the race.

It may sound cliche, but the race will be over before you know it. Don't just try to survive the race; aim to truly enjoy the race. You have put in the work. Now is the time to learn why Ultra Marathons are a coveted feat. During the race, it may be easy to start thinking about how far you have to go. However, I encourage you not to count down the miles but to stay in each moment.

Some people find it helpful to focus on an object in the distance and to make a short goal of running to that object. After reaching it, you find another distance object to make an interim goal to run to. Take time to enjoy nature using as many senses as possible. If you so choose, you can create a race day playlist. There are many running playlists online; however, if you do decide to have one, I would suggest spending the time to curate it just for you and possibly just for the race. What do you think you will need to hear at the first few checkpoints? In between checkpoints? Towards the end? Sometimes having external noise can help distract from the time left and any discomfort. It can also provide a way to enjoy the journey better.

Enjoy the Race

I encourage you to find joy in the pain and the mental battle. You may wonder how there can be joy when there is pain. Well, I believe the secret to this during the race is to have gratitude. Have gratitude for being able to make it to this point. For your body in carrying you this far even though you have and are pushing it to its limits. For your health. Be grateful for your support—the people cheering you on. Remember that our bodies were made to move and have the capacity to run beyond what you thought possible.

Running gives you the opportunity to enjoy nature. It exposes you to the world in various ways and forces you into a state where you become more aware of your surroundings. You begin to focus more on the rocks and trees that you climb over and fly past. You noticed people's faces, body posture, and demeanor. It's almost as if when you are running with the repetitive sound of your feet hitting the ground in a cadence, you enter into a spiritual awareness of yourself and your place in this world. While that might sound a little esoteric, it's true. Running, especially trail running, brings you into contact with nature that you wouldn't normally experience on a treadmill or in a gym. Ultra Marathons will often take place in locations that have a wide area to run. This is just more opportunity to experience nature at its best.

But it's not just about nature. Running, even when you're running with other people, is a solo and personal experience. The more you run, the more sights you will see and the more scenery you can enjoy. Never get so caught up in your running that you miss these beautiful moments. In a day and time where we are so caught up with being faster, more efficient, optimized, and measured by performance, running gives us a chance to slow down our minds and be more present in our current world. Even if you choose to use music or podcasts, you are still creating an environment in which you are indulging the core desire of your heart to get away and refocus. You create a zone where it's just you and the trail and whatever your mind is focused on. It's an experience worthy of a church.

Most of all, during your race, enjoy the fact that you are here. You made it. You put in the effort. You did the training. You are here because you chose to do the hard work and show up to this race. You have accomplished something here. As you run, whether by yourself or among a large group of people, remind yourself of that regularly. Take a moment to appreciate the moment and yourself for being here. This was no small feat.

Lastly, enjoy the feeling of doing what your body has been designed to do. Remember, we were made to run. Your body is now operating in its element. It's using the muscles, bones, tendons, and ligaments exactly how they were meant to be used. Feel the way that your body moves and strides along. Embrace the feeling of being active, out, and moving. Inhale and let your lungs respond to the efforts of your body. Enjoy your act of running.

7

CELEBRATE AND RECOVER

Perhaps it seems strange to have an entire chapter dedicated to celebration and recovery. It's such a small part of race preparation and execution. But the truth is that when your race ends, a new phase begins. What you do in the 24 to 72 hours after your race has a significant impact on not only your body but future races.

The moment that you cross the finish line, the race is finished. When that moment happens for you, I want you to take a beat to savor it. For the past several weeks and months, you have pushed your body to limits it hasn't seen before. You have spent time feeding and nourishing your body. You have spent time strengthening your mind. And the moment you cross that finish line, you realize it was all worth it.

Indulge and delight at this moment. No matter how you performed or how well you did or think you should've done, every race that you have trained, prepared for, and engaged in is a victory. There are people who could never even imagine thinking about completing an Ultra Marathon. The fact that you've even made it to the starting line puts you leagues ahead of others. But it's not really about celebrating how much better you are than other people. You made a commitment, put in the effort and work to achieve that commitment, and then put everything you had out there. Whether or not things went to plan—you are worthy of celebration.

CELEBRATE

After you finish your race, it's normal to have a range of emotions. For the person who has felt like they just reached an amazing goal that they worked so hard for, they may want to continue chasing that high. And who wouldn't? Nothing beats the feeling of being able to relish the satisfaction of personal victory. The temptation may be to stay in that feeling and find another race —to keep pushing and training. Some are surprised by how quickly after the race they have the desire to return.

On the other hand, not everyone who crosses the finish line is ecstatic about it. Some may be disappointed if the race didn't go as planned. Perhaps there was an unforeseen circumstance that arose the day of, or maybe an injury that held you back. For these people, crossing the finish line is not the happy victory they thought they would have. I call this "post-race blues." This feeling often compels the runner to start training again as soon as possible. It may also compel them to put off training to avoid the fear of failure or disappointment. The common thread in either of these scenarios is how you process the outcome of the race.

Remember that the outcome of the race doesn't define you. However, the way you react to the outcome is where character building takes place. If you're one of the people who have the desire to keep training right away, ask yourself why? What do you feel like you are missing at this moment that urgent training will fulfill? What would you be risking to fulfill that desire? Health? Time with family? Contentment? Take note of what you are feeling as you finish and in the days to come.

Celebration is important because whether or not you completed your race how you wanted, you put in the effort that needs to be recognized. Even if only by you. Celebrating allows you to affirm your efforts and motivate yourself to continue. Different runners have different ways they choose to celebrate. Some people even have rituals—eating at the same restaurant or going out for the same drink after every successful race.

One very popular way that race finishers tend to celebrate is the tried-and-true method of eating your favorite food afterward. There's nothing like allowing yourself to let go after months of training on an intentional nutrition plan. After a big race, you'll be starving, and a plate of tasty food at a restaurant is a great way to finish off your day.

Travel is another way that many runners like to celebrate the completion of their race. Many Ultra Marathon runners will schedule vacation or travel experiences to allow them the chance to get away from the focused environment they have spent the last few months dwelling in. People use travel to clear their minds and to let off steam. After you have been running the same trail over and over and over for hours, you really just want to see something new. Traveling also fits in with this theme of going from point A to point B. And that's what running does. It takes you from point A to point B. So by choosing to celebrate the end of your race with travel, you are continuing the experience in a more relaxed manner, hopefully.

What is a celebration without friendship however? When you finish the race, it feels great to spend time with people you love and who love you. This doesn't even need to be a giant party. Sometimes, just knowing that there are people waiting for you at the end of the race and are talking about the high and low points on the ride back home is enough of a celebration. Sometimes hanging out afterwards and getting a smoothie or a drink can add to the excitement of finishing. Spending time with your loved ones also gives you the opportunity to hear positive feedback outside of your own head. If things didn't go according to plan or if you did not achieve the time that you wanted, hearing the encouragement and support from other people draws you outside of your own mind and into reality. Sometimes the best voices we can hear are the voices of those who understand and love us.

On the other hand, sometimes celebration can be found in just silently soaking in the moment. Maybe your celebration is going for a slow and steady walk in a park nearby. Taking deep breaths and soaking in the moment is just as much a celebration as screaming and yelling and whooping and hollering. Silent meditation can help you to appreciate and develop gratitude for all that you've just accomplished. Couple this with some journaling about your feelings directly afterwards, and you've got a solid record of the events of this important day.

Another form of celebration is to pamper yourself. This doesn't mean that you have to go out to an expensive spa and let people cater to your every need, although that sounds amazing. You can pamper yourself just by coming home, drawing a bath, making sure your bed is completely comfortable, setting out a plate of your favorite food, whether you prepare yourself or get it from a restaurant, playing your favorite music, and allowing yourself to just be. After soaking in your tub, allowing your muscles to relax, and eating your favorite food while watching a movie you love, you can finish off the night by slipping into your comfy bed and allowing yourself to drift off into peaceful bliss.

Playing games is also a form of celebration. After using your body to its utmost limits, spending a couple of days burying yourself in a new video game or playing board games with friends can be a great way to acknowledge your hard work and allow yourself to rest. Coincidentally, it can also serve as a great motivator when you're in the middle of a run to know that all you have to do is get through this challenge, and then you get the chance to relax.

Celebration comes in many different forms. However you choose to celebrate, make sure that you allow yourself time to acknowledge that all your hard work was worth it.

REST AND RECOVER

Oftentimes while you run, due to the endorphins and focus, you may not notice minor irritants or sores. After cooling down, take a few moments to inspect for any blisters, cuts, and tender areas with swelling. If there is a medic, you could stop by to have a second set of eyes check you out.

As tempting as it may be, avoid taking NSAIDs like ibuprofen, Aleve, etc. While these medications can help with the inflammation likely coursing throughout your body, they can also affect your kidney function. Your kidneys need to get adequate blood flow, and the effects of muscle breakdown may also affect them. Staying hydrated and avoiding these medications are one of the best ways you can support your kidney health after the race. If you need some pain relief, Tylenol may be the best option, but talk with the medic at the site for their recommendations.

In the absence of medication, one of the most common methods to reduce inflammation and help with tender muscles is the use of ice baths or cold showers. These can help reduce blood flow and the dispersion of heat throughout your body. They also have a cooling and soothing effect on your system overall.

There are some other ways to reduce inflammation. One of them is through diet. Turmeric, garlic, ginger, berries, tomatoes, nuts, and leafy greens are all known to help fight inflammation in the body. Omega 3 fatty acids are also an excellent nutrient that helps promote recovery. Algae is an excellent source of omega-three fatty acids for those who are plant-based. If you are not plant-based but aren't a fan of seafood, you can also take it in the form of a supplement. Omega-three fatty acids also help with recovery by decreasing inflammation in the body. It is also good for your heart and your eyes.

I recommend taking vitamin C supplements and immunity boosters following the race. One study found that 33-68% of Ultra Marathon runners will experience an upper respiratory infection in the two weeks following the race. This finding is not particularly surprising, and it has been suggested that stress hormones which are known to weaken the immune system when released over a long period of time, may be one of the reasons for this. Your body has been under extreme amounts of stress—and if this is your first race, more than it probably ever has been. You wouldn't recommend to a friend that they still go to work when they are still running a fever from the flu; similarly, if you find yourself feeling under the weather, give yourself rest and all the home remedies. Even if you don't fall ill, it's important to allow space to recover due to possibly having a weakened immune system.

Reducing inflammation and caring for injury is only one part of dealing with recovery and rest after your race. There are several other things that you can do in order to maximize recovery and healing. Your goal should be for your body to reach equilibrium as soon as possible, as safe as possible. The following are a few concepts you should keep in mind during your recovery period.

Stay Active

After you cross the finish line, there may be a temptation to collapse on the ground like spaghetti and layout. Resist that urge. Bring yourself to a slow stop and keep walking. It may take up to 30 minutes to cool down. This will allow your body to gradually lower your heart rate and body temperature. It is important that you remain hydrated even after the race. As you have been losing salt through sweat, it would be best to drink fluids that will replace those electrolytes. There are also oral rehydration products you can purchase, which include salts and glucose.

You should also take some time to eat a simple snack, even if you plan on eating a much larger dinner at a restaurant later. Eating a simple bagel or some trail mix helps to give your body energy for that post-exercise burn that happens as your metabolism continues long after your body has stopped. You can also have some protein bars that have a large percentage of carbohydrates included.

This is also an excellent time to change into comfortable shoes and clothes. Part of being active is being comfortable and allowing yourself to rest in that feeling. You may also want to get out of your sweaty clothes sooner rather than later to keep from getting cold or to decrease the risk of chafing. Changing your clothes also helps to remind you to stay active and serves as an excellent way to focus on something other than flopping down and going to sleep.

Make sure to stretch and restore motion to your poor muscles, which have been working overtime for the past few hours. No matter what you do, you have to keep moving and staying mobile. Some good stretches you should make sure to complete during this time include quads and hamstrings stretches as well as your torso. Take these stretches slow so as to prevent injury. These are cooldown stretches, not warm-up stretches, so be gentle with yourself; your muscles have just put in a lot of time and effort.

Performing some yoga after taking a breather post-Ultra Marathon is a great way to get the blood moving, stretch out your limbs, and allow your body to cool down slowly and in a controlled manner. You might also consider massaging or foam rolling to squeeze out the lactic acid and keep the muscles supple. This helps keep the muscles from getting stiff and tightening up on you. It can also help prevent cramps.

Allow for Sleep

It's not uncommon for runners to have difficulty sleeping after a long and intense race, despite the fatigue that seems to dwell in their very bones. In fact, many runners complain of post-race insomnia and become anxious at the thought of their body being unwilling to recover because they cannot get good sleep. This sensation does fade over time. Running a race is a full-body sensory extravaganza. Our thoughts are in overdrive; our nose is smelling food, sweat, and the aroma of nature. Our ears are listening to the sound of our breath, the pattering of feet on the ground, and the cheers of spectators. Our mouth is dry or pacing the snacks or water and electrolytes we are chugging into our system. Our body feels the wind as air presses against us, the sensation of our feet hitting the ground rhythmically, the sweat on our face and arms, and of course, the sensation of the full-body mechanics moving in unison. Our eyes are watching the ground in front of us, the people around us, and the scenic views we are passing by. Running is a full-body experience. Your brain needs time to process that.

Sleep is how our body heals. After your Ultra Marathon, you must take time to rest and sleep. Even if you don't feel like sleeping, make sure to allow for that time. This may mean you need to add a few extra hours to your sleep plan. That's okay; your body will thank you later.

But sleep is not just for your body; it's also for your mind. You have been mentally focused on one goal for hours on end. Even if your mind wanders, there are always the underlying thoughts that are playing their way through as you plan your course, think about what you're going to do next, and focus on keeping your pace. You have strained your mind in order to optimize your body. Give your mind a chance to process and relax. Your consciousness is full of images of the trail as well as the sensation of your feet hitting the ground over and over and over.

Although I am recommending that you sleep as much as you can, it's okay if you can't sleep as well. Some-times your mind may still be racing, or you may naturally be unable to sleep for long periods of time. That's okay; this is only one aspect of the rest and recovery phase of your Ultra Marathon journey. Often this difficulty with sleep can be due to an elevated body temperature. Our body temperature naturally cools when we go to sleep, and sometimes when our body is having trouble cooling down, it can make sleep hard to capture. Making sure you're adequately hydrated can help offset this.

Take Time Off

As a general rule, when trying to figure out the best timeline, you should allow yourself one day to recover for every hour you spent racing. You may even consider taking a few days off from work following the race, depending on the nature of your job. I can't emphasize enough how important it is to take it easy. Out of habit, you may want to get back into the same routine. I'm not saying to be a couch potato the next two weeks unless that's truly what you feel like your body needs.

Perhaps, however, you can hold off on high-intensity training for two weeks. Allow your body the chance to reset. If you're feeling antsy, you can go on simple, leisurely walks. No hard exercise. During those walks, you can take time to meditate or regroup. You can reflect on the race and process. It doesn't matter what you choose to do, as long as you are not doing any intensive exercise during this time.

Refusing to take time off after a marathon can lead to injuries and overtraining. Without a chance to heal, your muscles can actually become weaker and your body less stable. Your body is more at risk than ever after an intense race. The same goes for your immune system. Without adequate rest, your system can become fatigued, and you can have the same effects as if you hadn't slept for a few days or stayed outside in the cold for too long.

Let's address the elephant in the room.

Fear.

Most runners don't take time off because they're afraid of losing their current level of fitness. The idea of skipping training and suffering a loss in fitness level is agitating. Let's nip this fear in the bud. Yes, you will suffer some minor loss to your fitness level. Yes, you will have to train to get that back. But I guarantee you that you will lose even more of your fitness if you suffer an injury because of overtraining and have to keep off your leg for a month.

Take your time and wait a few weeks before doing any significant race training again. Use that time to improve your technique and try some different (lighter) activities. Or you can use that time to look ahead to the future and plan what you'll do when you get back into training.

WHAT'S NEXT?

After the race, it can be helpful for some people to debrief or process with either a coach, a trusted friend, or on your own. If this is your first big race and you may be new to some of the different emotions that you may be feeling. It can be easy to keep dwelling on the race, replaying each part over and over in your head. Setting aside time will allow you to be able to better organize your thoughts.

Some questions to consider include things like: What are three things that went well? What were some things that surprised you before, during, or after the race? What is one thing that you would change or do differently? Yes, just one thing. It's so much easier, and it's human nature to focus more on the negative than the positive. And the negative is what tends to stick in our minds the most. So during this processing time, we want to rewire our brains a bit so that we remember the positive aspects of the race and therefore are more likely to continue and repeat the good aspects. And what are some things that you are grateful for about your race?

144 | THE ULTRA MARATHON BIBLE

After you feel you have adequately rested, you will likely want to start planning for your next race. If you just ran your first 50k, after your recovery, you might consider setting a goal to run 50m. If you just ran 50m, then perhaps set your eyes towards 100k. Or from a 100k to 100m. When thinking about your next race, you might feel the excitement, but it can also feel over-whelming. Remember that when setting goals, it can be helpful to make them SMART. That is, Specific, Measurable, Attainable, Relevant, and Time-frame. Basically, if you just ran a 50k, as much as you might want to run a 100m, that may not be as realistic or attainable. However, it's certainly a goal you can work up to while setting smaller goals in between.

LEAVE A 1-CLICK REVIEW!

Customer reviews

★★★★★ 5 out of 5

5 global ratings

5 star		100%
4 star		0%
3 star		0%
2 star		0%
1 star		0%

⌄ How customer reviews and ratings work

Review this product

Share your thoughts with other customers

Write a customer review

I would be incredibly thankful if you could take just 60 seconds to write a brief review on Amazon, even if it's just a few sentences

Scan the QR code below to leave your review.

CONCLUSION

By now, you should have a good idea of everything that it takes to complete an Ultra Marathon. This is not an impossible task. People do it all the time. With proper training, preparation, and execution, you can also have the amazing experience of running and completing an Ultra Marathon.

Everything contained in these pages is a guide for your individual journey. While following it will allow you to develop healthy practices and set you on the right path, every runner's journey is unique. Feel free to take some of the information and leave the rest. You were made to run, and if you take the time to explore this art, I believe you'll see that as well.

Remember that you are entering into a world made up of an amazing community. There are men and women who have been running much longer than you who can share their experiences and strength. They have a lot of advice and knowledge to offer if you're willing to listen and receive it. All you have to do is ask. Don't be afraid of getting involved and growing your community. If you're a runner, you're one of us.

One of the cool things about learning to participate in an Ultra Marathon is that you now have the tools to prepare for any race. From this point forward, the only thing limiting you is your own willingness. Whether you're looking to improve your running strategies or learn new ones for the first time ever, there is a whole world out there. Run in exciting places, meet interesting people, and explore this amazing sport. Challenge yourself and continue to grow. And no matter how difficult the race, remember that you were made to run. You now know how to get started, so get running.

I'll see you on the trail.

CUSTOMIZABLE TRAINING PLANS
PROVIDED BELOW

For 50K, 50M, 100K, & 100M

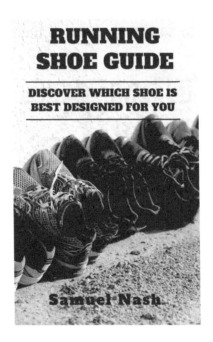

This running shoe guide goes into detail about the many different types of running shoes, and which one is the best fit for you.

REFERENCES

Andrews, M. (2021, August 16). *What Is Ultra Running? Ultramarathons, Explained.* Marathon Handbook. https://marathonhandbook.com/what-is-ultra-running/

ASFA. (n.d.). *Running Ultra Marathons - The Benefits of Having a Crew and Pacers.* ASFA. Retrieved May 28, 2022, from https://www.americansportandfitness.com/blogs/fitness-blog/running-ultra-marathons-the-benefits-of-having-a-crew-and-pacers#:~:text=Having%20a%20crew%20helps%20cut

Bakkala, A. (2019, November 13). *Tips for Your First Ultramarathon.* ACTIVE.com. https://www.active.com/running/articles/tips-for-your-first-ultramarathon

Blow, A. (2021, July 14). *Sweat Testing 101.* Triathlete. https://www.triathlete.com/nutrition/sweat-testing-101/

Burfoot, A. (2001, November 14). *The 10-Percent Rule.* Runner's World. https://www.runnersworld.com/training/a20781512/the-10-percent-rule/#:~:text=The%2010%2Dpercent%20rule%20

Carrier, D. R., Kapoor, A. K., Kimura, T., Nickels, M. K., Scott, E. C., So, J. K., & Trinkaus, E. (1984). The Energetic Paradox of Human Running and Hominid Evolution [and Comments and Reply]. *Current Anthropology, 25*(4), 483–495. https://doi.org/10.1086/203165

Cederborg, J. (2006, October 5). *Pass The Salt?* Runner's World. https://www.runnersworld.com/nutrition-weight-loss/a20784078/pass-the-salt/

Clarke, M. (2012, September 30). *6 Fun Facts About Ultrarunning.* Active.com. https://www.active.com/running/articles/6-fun-facts-about-ultrarunning

Costa, R. J. S., Knechtle, B., Tarnopolsky, M., & Hoffman, M. D. (2019). Nutrition for Ultramarathon Running: Trail, Track, and Road.

International Journal of Sport Nutrition and Exercise Metabolism, 29(2), 130–140. https://doi.org/10.1123/ijsnem.2018-0255

D'Aulerio, M. (2017, April 7). *11 Things To Consider Before Signing Up For An Ultra Marathon - Long Run Living.* Long Run Living. http://www.longrunliving.com/11-things-to-consider-before-signing-up-for-an-ultra-marathon/

Davis, N. (2021, October 11). *Is Running Bad for Your Knees?* Healthline. https://www.healthline.com/health/fitness/is-running-bad-for-your-knees#what-the-science-says

Gluck, W. (Director). (2014, December 7). *Annie* [Film]. Columbia Pictures, Village Roadshow Pictures, Sony Pictures Releasing.

Higdon, H. (2020). *MARATHON : the ultimate training guide - advice,plans, and programs for half and full marat.* Rodale.

Kenefick, R. W. (2018). Drinking Strategies: Planned Drinking Versus Drinking to Thirst. *Sports Medicine, 48*(S1), 31–37. https://doi.org/10.1007/s40279-017-0844-6

Laney, D. (2019, June 25). *An Introduction to Crewing.* IRunFar. https://www.irunfar.com/an-introduction-to-crewing

Lash, J. P. (1997). *Helen and teacher : the story of Helen Keller and Anne Sullivan Macy.* Addison-Wesley.

Mcdougall, C. (2016). *Born to run : a hidden tribe, superathletes, and the greatest race the world has never seen.* Alfred A. Knopf.

McMillan, G. (2016, September 27). *THE RUNNER'S GUIDE TO ICE BATHS.* McMillan Running. https://www.mcmillanrunning.com/the-runners-guide-to-ice-baths/

Peter, L. J. (1977). *Peter's quotations : ideas for our time.* Bantam Books.

Rom, Z. (2020, April 24). *Gearing Up For Your First Ultramarathon.* Trail Runner Magazine. https://www.trailrunnermag.com/gear/accessories-gear/gearing-up-for-your-first-ultramarathon/

Runningforthehills20. (2021, June 11). *How Long Should I Rest After an Ultra Marathon? - Running for the Hills.* Running for the Hills. https://runningforthehills.com/resting-after-an-ultra-marathon

Russell, S. (2019, January 8). *Best Training Advice for a New Ultramarathon Runner.* Runners Connect. https://runnersconnect.net/first-ultra-runner-questions/

Smart, D. (2022, April 25). *Why you don't need to hydrate on short runs.* Canadian Running Magazine. https://runningmagazine.ca/sections/training/why-you-dont-need-to-hydrate-on-short-runs/

Tocci, K. (2021, October 18). *How To Run 100 Miles: Essential Training Guide + Training Plan.* Marathonhandbook.com. https://marathonhandbook.com/how-to-run-100-mile-training-plan/

Wainwright, A., & Derry Brabbs. (1996). *Wainwright's coast to coast walk.* Michael Joseph.

Made in United States
Cleveland, OH
14 November 2024

10668389R00085